New England Deaconess Hospital

A Century of Caring

Carl M. Brauer

Library of Congress Catalog Card Number: 95–71694

ISBN 0–9649135–0–X

Designed by Kohn Cruikshank Inc, Boston;
Typeset in Monotype Bembo and Adobe Frutiger
on a Macintosh Computer;
The paper is Simpson Vicksburg Starwhite Archiva
vellum finish text;
Printed in Hong Kong by Palace Press International.

P R E F A C E

FOUNDED BY METHODIST DEACONESSES to serve missionary purposes, the New England Deaconess Hospital opened its doors in Boston in 1896 as a modest fourteen-bed hospital with only rudimentary equipment. Today a more secular institution, the Deaconess occupies a cluster of modern buildings with nearly 400 beds, extensive outpatient services, and the latest in sophisticated medical technology and patient care. Located in the midst of one of the world's great hospital and medical complexes, the Deaconess is a tertiary-care, specialty-referral hospital, a major teaching affiliate of Harvard Medical School, and home to substantial and important research.

Obviously, the Deaconess of 1996 is a very different place from the Deaconess of 1896. Yet, there are also certain important continuities between then and now, most especially in the high-quality and sensitive patient care which lies at the heart of the Deaconess's institutional culture. Within twenty years of the hospital's founding, clinical scientific investigations were under way, and within forty years of its opening, specialty training and fellowships had been established, as well as loose ties to Harvard Medical School. Thus, the seeds of today's Deaconess were planted and cultivated early, both at the hospital's founding and in its first four decades.

The Deaconess commissioned this history as part of its centennial celebration. At earlier benchmarks, both the hospital and its affiliated school of nursing published histories that proved valuable in the preparation of this book. This marks the first time, however, that the hospital asked an independent, profes-sional historian to undertake the job of writing its story. My assignment was to write an objective, readable, and engaging institutional history and that is what I hope to have produced.

When recording the annals of any institution, it helps to have an interesting cast of characters through whom the story can be told. This I have had in abundance at the Deaconess. Its cast includes many dedicated, accomplished, and interesting individuals, among them Mary Lunn, Adeliza Betts, Maurice Howe Richardson, Elliott Joslin, Frank Lahey, Shields Warren, Leland McKittrick, Richard Overholt, F. Gorham Brigham, Warren Cook, Lyman Hoyt, Ellen Howland, and Don Lowry. And the more contemporary cast is every bit as good.

I pay some attention to the larger historical context of which the Deaconess was a part in order to understand how the hospital fits into a larger picture. In so doing, I have drawn upon the history of medicine, hospitals, and nursing, and of Boston and the United States. But my assignment was not to produce a "life and times" of the Deaconess. Rather, I was asked to focus primarily on the hospital itself, paying somewhat disproportionate attention to the most recent fifty years. The intended audience for this history is the extended Deaconess family, which numbers in the thousands — current and former staff, patients, trustees and corporators, volunteers, friends, and donors. Those who lack an immediate connection to the Deaconess may also find this book worthwhile, particularly if they are interested in medical, hospital, and nursing history generally, and specifically, in the history of medical institutions in Boston.

This volume treats certain sensitive topics and controversies in the hospital's history, including ones that occurred in the relatively recent past. Although it would have been easy to skip over controversies and avoid unpleasant details, that would have resulted in a dishonest and incomplete story, which would have deservedly lacked credibility. It would also have been easy for me to become a partisan in disagreements or to sit in judgment of certain practices or individuals. But I did not feel those would be appropriate roles for me to play. Nor did I think they would enhance the book's value.

While a number of individuals at the Deaconess, from both the active and retired staffs, have read the manuscript in progress, no one has altered the essence of what I have written. Most of the comments I received on preliminary drafts were on style or involved questions of fact and accuracy, not interpretation. So, I am the sole author of this history; any errors of omission or commission are mine alone. Readers may well disagree with my version or interpretation of events or with the relative weight I have accorded certain developments or individuals, but I hope they will feel that I have tried to be objective, accurate, and fair.

I have had full access to the hospital's older existing records, with the exception of patient files, which are, of course, confidential. Many of the hospital's records are now located in an archive in the Gilbert Horrax Library. I also benefited from unlimited access to board minutes, which are housed in the legal counsel's office, and papers of the New England Deaconess Hospital School of Nursing, which are on deposit at the Bapst Library at Boston College. In addition, I drew upon published materials at the Francis A. Countway Library of Medicine, the Harry Elkins Widener Library, and the Andover-Harvard Library, all at Harvard University.

Interviews with selected participants in the Deaconess's history as well as with a few key observers constituted a major and invaluable primary source. These several dozen interviews were conducted over a three-year period. Sadly, several of those I interviewed have since died. I have generally avoided quoting directly from interviews since they were not formal oral histories — my subjects never had the opportunity to correct the record. But I have taken the liberty of quoting from them briefly on occasion when I felt confident that the quotations would add color without proving embarrassing to anyone. I have deposited the tapes of these interviews as well as my notes in the Deaconess archive.

Researching and writing this book has been a pleasure, both because the subject was fascinating and because virtually everyone I dealt with was kind, helpful, and forthcoming. It would be impossible to acknowledge all of those who helped bring this book to fruition, but I would be remiss if I did not specifically acknowledge and thank a number of especially helpful contributors.

In writing an institution's history, it is invaluable to have support and involvement from the organization's leader, and I have had them both in abundance from Dick Gaintner. His belief in the importance of history was responsible for initiating this project. Despite his extremely busy schedule, he made time to read and comment on chapter drafts and the completed manuscript. I have, moreover, been triply fortunate in that Laurie MacLure and Don Lowry, Gaintner's predecessors as the Deaconess's chief executive, have also been firmly behind this project. Laurie and Don were always available to answer questions and to provide good leads, and they, too, were scrupulous and tactful readers of individual chapter drafts.

With grace, humor, and tact, George Starkey chaired a history advisory committee at the Deaconess, becoming my friend in the process. Serving faithfully alongside him were Laurie MacLure, Jim Tullis, Bill McDermott, and Judy Miller. At the Deaconess, I also received helpful feedback on later chapters from Bob Moellering, Glenn Steele, Mel Clouse, and Harvey Goldman. In addition, I benefited enormously from the comments of two outside readers of the manuscript in progress: Allan M. Brandt, the Amalie Moses Kass Professor of the History of Medicine at Harvard Medical School; and Richard J. Wolfe, Curator of Rare Books and Manuscripts at the Francis A. Countway Library of Medicine at Harvard Medical School.

Roger Perry was throughout a highly knowledgeable and efficient liaison and problem solver for me at the Deaconess. Paul Vaiginas and Diane Young were welcoming and helpful at the Horrax Library as were Barbara Kellman in the legal counsel's office and Pamela Lawrence and Lisa Kushnir in the Office of Communications. Dennis Scott of the John J. Burns Library at Boston College assisted in providing access to the photographic archives of the New England Deaconess School of Nursing as did Madeleine W. Mullin in the Countway Library. Judy Kohn created an elegant design that reflects the form and substance of the Deaconess story. Susan Pasternack did a first-rate job managing the details of publication, as well as contributing photo research and selection, caption writing, and editing.

To all of the above and many others who are not named here, I am deeply grateful. I hope this book justifies the confidence that many people have shown in me and in this project.

Carl M. Brauer

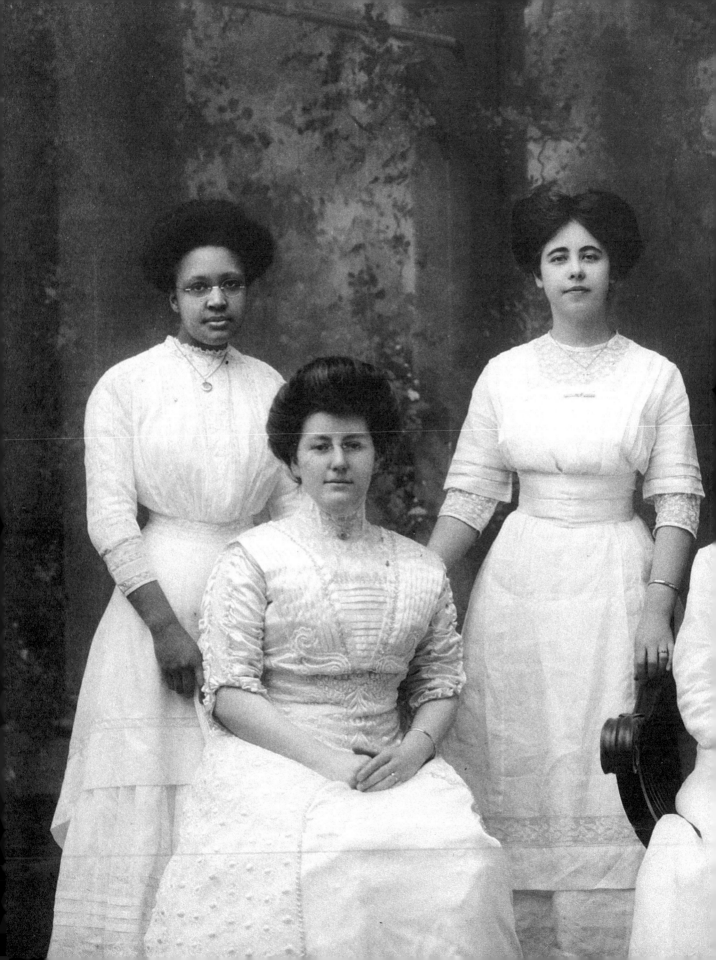

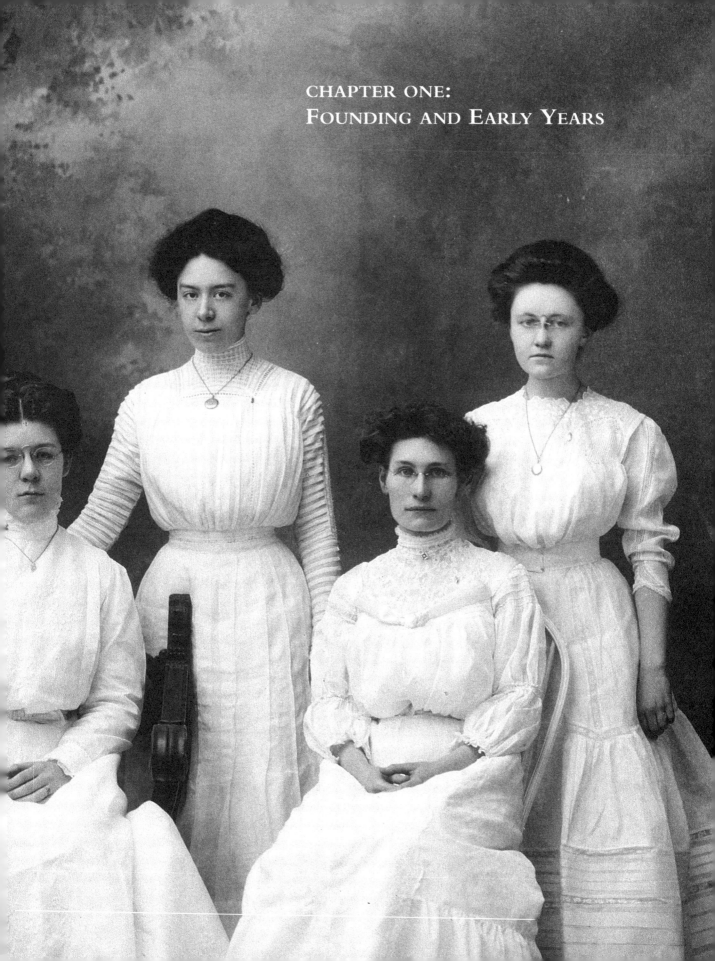

Overleaf:

Graduates of the New England Deaconess Training School, May 1911. Described in contemporary accounts as "ministering angels," the early Methodist deaconesses and trainees established an enduring legacy of providing competent and compassionate care. Deaconesses fulfilled important community services that ranged from missionary work to teaching and nursing. Graduates of the religious program interested in professional nursing practice often continued their studies at the Nurses' Training School. In time the program of religious studies moved to Boston University while the hospital continued to support a fully professional and secular hospital-based nurse training school.

Standing (left to right):
Cora Scott, Pearl B. Gosnell, Charlotte M. Leusher, Addie A. Crocke

Seated (left to right):
Ella W. Hunter, Audrey L. Hunt, Maude C. Andrews

CHAPTER ONE:
FOUNDING AND EARLY YEARS

New England Deaconess Hospital opened its doors in a five-story Boston brownstone in 1896, with one foot planted solidly in the nineteenth century and the other reaching gingerly toward the twentieth. The hospital's founding coincided with profound changes that were beginning to transform hospitals, medical science, and nursing. In its early years, New England Deaconess Hospital inevitably underwent significant change as well, establishing its own distinctive values and culture while making a mark in Boston and the larger world.

'A MODEL OF ITS KIND'

Throughout history, hospitals were essentially charities that served a poor and dependent population. In both purpose and practice, little separated them from almshouses. When sickness struck members of the middle and upper classes, they generally chose to be cared for at home rather than in hospitals, which were stigmatized and feared. Because of medical advances, however, particularly in surgery, hospitals became a plausible if not desirable alternative to home care in the decades preceding the First World War. Thus, many new institutions were established and existing ones expanded. The use of ether as an anesthetic and the adoption of asepsis in the surgical environment enhanced both the possibilities and safety of surgery. Private, middle-class patients, who were charged for bed, board, and services, began to fill hospital beds, providing an economic base not formerly enjoyed. Hospitals simultaneously became much more central to medical practice itself; for doctors, and especially for surgeons, access became critical.

By 1910 there were more than 4,000 hospitals in the United States. It has been estimated that over 80 percent of these private and voluntary institutions had been established during the preceding thirty years. Hospitals were classified as either specialty or general, with ownership falling into one of three categories: proprietary; private voluntary, often with a sectarian affiliation; and public — municipal, county, or state. The line between public and private *purpose* was often blurred, however; voluntary hospitals, for example, frequently accepted patients who could pay only part or none of their bills.

Like many institutions founded in these years, New England Deaconess Hospital had sectarian roots, in its case, Methodist. A Protestant evangelical movement begun by John Wesley in eighteenth-century England, Methodism had subsequently been transported to the American colonies. Methodists believed in personal and social morality, in the perfectibility of man, and in applied Christianity. Methodist missionaries had found fertile soil in the colonies and then in the young states — in 1780, there were 8,500 adherents in America; ten years later that number had grown sevenfold.

The denomination continued to expand at a rapid rate through the nineteenth century, founding or controlling numerous colleges and universities in the United States. At the same time, American Methodism suffered schisms and other divisions and separated into white southern and black churches. Taken together, however, in 1900 the five and a half million Methodists constituted the largest Protestant denomination in the United States. (Baptists surpassed Methodists in numbers in the 1920s.)

The Methodist Episcopal Church (northern), the largest branch of Methodism, was home in the 1880s to a deaconess movement which traced its origins to Germany. There, in Kaiserwerth in the 1830s, Theodor Fliedner, a Lutheran pastor, along with his wife, Friederike, had established a small refuge for discharged prisoners. The Fliedners later added an orphanage, a normal school, and a small hospital staffed by deaconesses, religious women who modeled themselves on early Christian ideals. The deaconesses were not the first to take up the cause: Catholic sisterhoods, such as the Sisters of Charity, the Sisters of Mercy, and the Sisters of the Holy Cross, it should be noted, had been involved in founding and running hospitals well before their Protestant counterparts.

One of those influenced by the work of the Fliedners was Florence Nightingale, a well-born Englishwoman who heeded a religious calling to become a nurse. Inspired by what she saw and experienced in Kaiserwerth in 1850 and 1851, Nightingale devoted herself to the profession and subsequently became famous for her heroic work with the British army during the Crimean War. Known as the "lady with the lamp," Nightingale went on to found modern nursing, becoming an influential crusader for improved, hygienic hospitals and for professional nursing training.

In time the deaconess movement spread to the Methodist Church throughout Germany and England, and eventually to America. The first

Methodist home and training school for deaconesses in the United States was established in Chicago in 1887. The following year a second institution opened in Cincinnati, along with a hospital managed by deaconesses. Several other cities soon followed suit, including Boston.

In April 1889, the New England Conference of Methodists, an affiliate of the Methodist Episcopal Church, recommended the establishment of a deaconess home and training school in Boston or vicinity, appropriating $150 for that purpose and appointing the Reverend William Nast Brodbeck as head of a special committee to make the necessary arrangements. Isabella Thoburn, who had been housemother in Chicago, aided in the organization. Seven months later, in November 1889, the New England Home and Training School opened at 45 East Chester Park (693 Massachusetts Avenue) in Boston. Previously a private residence, the site had been purchased by the New England Conference of Methodists for $7,600, financed in significant part by a mortgage. Prior to opening, an additional $1,000 was spent on repairs. Through contributions, however, the home was able to retire its debt by 1891.

Appointed the first superintendent of the New England Home and Training School was Mary E. Lunn, a Chicago-trained deaconess. Although diminutive in stature, Lunn was indefatigable in spirit. "We do not accept any candidates under 23 or more than 40 years of age," she told a reporter soon after her arrival. "They must furnish satisfactory recommendations from their pastors and the official boards of the churches to which they belong and present a health certificate from a physician. The office of deaconess is not a sinecure, and the church cannot afford to train any who have not the health, as well as the spirit, for successful service."

During that first year, the new home accommodated ten women besides Lunn, including a deaconess and several candidates. Within a few years, the number of trainees, who came primarily from New England, had grown so rapidly that additional space had to be rented to house them all. Those accepted for admission agreed "to abide by the decisions of the Superintendent, cheerfully giving all their time to the work assigned them. Candidates are desired to furnish, if possible, their own bedding, especially blankets." Both probationers and deaconesses were permitted to pay for their own board and

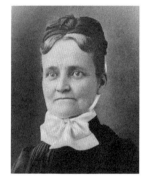

MARY E. LUNN, CA. 1896.
A Chicago-trained deaconess who was sent on a temporary basis to help launch the New England Home and Training School, Lunn remained eleven years and served as the first superintendent of both the home and training school and New England Deaconess Hospital. She brought great energy, vision, and devotion to helping establish the hospital.

expenses, though the home provided them if necessary; the women received no salary.

The requirements for ordination included a minimum of two years of study and work and candidates had to be at least twenty-five years old. When women were ordained, they were presumed to be entering their life's work, although no irrevocable vow was required. Methodist deaconesses were proud of the public ceremony that commemorated ordination, where all could hear their vows and the church's covenant to them. In nineteenth-century America the secretiveness of Catholic sisterhoods had given rise to fears and even hysteria among Protestants.

The early work of the Boston deaconesses was primarily missionary in nature. "One frequently meets upon the streets, and especially in those crowded and poverty-stricken districts where sin, suffering and sickness prevail, quiet, unassuming women garbed in black and wearing plain gray bonnets," reported the *Boston Globe*. "The 'gray bonnets,' as they are sometimes dubbed by the poor people who look eagerly for their coming are deaconesses of the Methodist Episcopal church." Reflecting Methodism's emphasis on sweetness and warmth, the deaconesses distributed hundreds of bouquets of flowers. An early history explained, "The duties of the deaconess are to minister to the poor, visit the sick, pray with the dying, care for the orphans, seek the wandering, comfort the sorrowing, save the sinning, and relinquishing all other pursuits, she is to devote herself, in a general way, to such forms of Christian labor as may be suited to her abilities."

From the start, however, Lunn envisaged opening a hospital, an orphan asylum, a home for the aged, and "social reformatories" in addition to the home and training school. As the Cincinnati experience indicated, Methodist deaconesses had already established hospitals elsewhere. Other religious orders had opened several in Boston. The Sisters of St. Margaret, an Anglican order, constituted the original nursing staff at Children's Hospital and then founded their own dispensary and hospital, while Carney Hospital was owned and operated by the Catholic Sisters of Charity.

In her report of 1893, Lunn outlined the specific advantages that would accrue from opening even a very small facility. Principally, she noted, it would allow her to hire hospital-trained nurses to instruct students in the care of the sick. "We should soon have workers whom we could send out to do efficient service for those who are often found by our visiting deaconesses with absolutely no one to care for them, and I am convinced that if this part of our work were emphasized it would appeal more directly to the sympathies of the public, and thus secure a more cordial support." According to the superintendent, the establishment of a hospital would enhance the deaconesses' reputation and facilitate their missionary work.

The hospital had to be postponed, however. As Rev. Brodbeck, who had become president of the Deaconess Association's Board of Managers, explained two years later, the group was unable to find a suitable location and the economic depression (of 1893) made it inadvisable to assume any further financial obligation. Though severe, the depression abated fairly quickly, however, and soon the corporation empowered the Board of Managers to pursue the expansion plan once again. "We are satisfied that our deaconess work in Boston and vicinity can never reach its highest efficiency until we have a Hospital in successful operation," the Board of Managers declared in its report of 1894–95. According to a short hospital history published in 1940, a committee was formed in 1894 "to plan a hospital where science and Christian kindliness should unite in combating disease," though these exact words do not appear in the original surviving records.

In 1900 an Association report set forth the goals for the new undertaking: "The object of the New England Deaconess Hospital is to afford those who need and desire it an opportunity to avail themselves of the skill of the most eminent physicians and surgeons in New England, and at the same time enjoy the comforts of a home where the very atmosphere seems laden with that warmth and sweetness of devotion which makes pain more easily borne, and which hastens the return of health." The second aim, the report continued, was to "train young women" who would give their lives to nursing, "especially as deaconesses, either in the hospital (after their course of training is completed) or in district nursing among the poor."

Seeking to create a homelike atmosphere, New England Deaconess Hospital began its operations in what had once been a residence: a five-story, fourteen-room brownstone purchased by the Board of Managers for $8,000 at 691 Massachusetts Avenue adjacent to the New England Home and Training School. Although inadequate in both design and space, the building was all the Association could afford and at least had the advantage of being conveniently located. On February 5, 1896, more than 100 people gathered in the rain for the dedication of the little fourteen-bed infirmary.

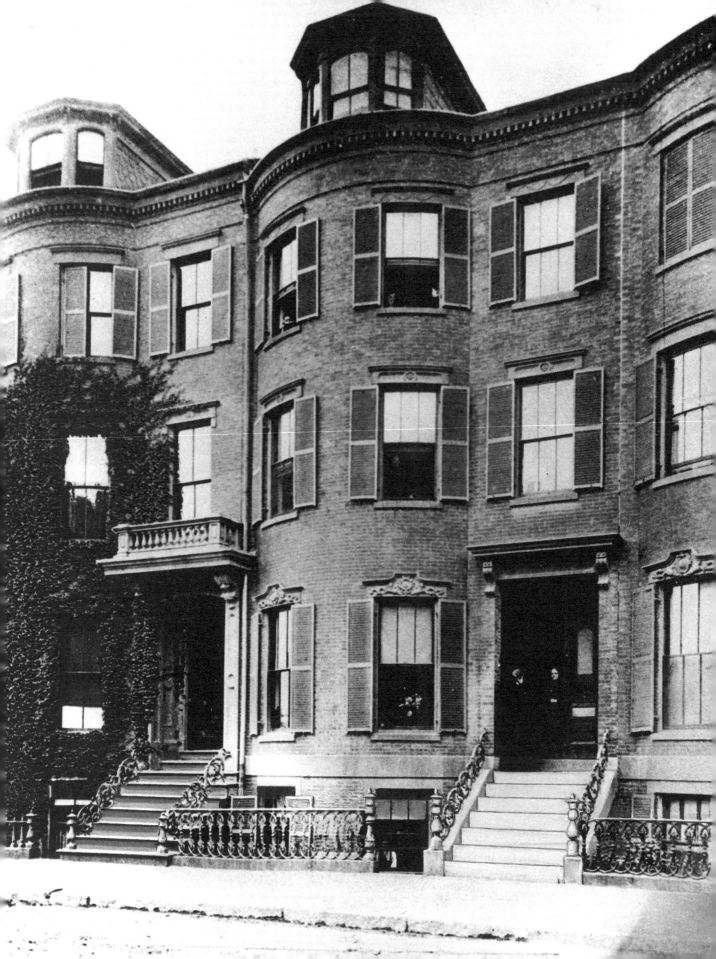

Money and resources were scarce at the start and the hospital had to depend upon the generosity of its neighbors and supporters. For the first several months, the hospital lacked a telephone, relying instead on one belonging to a doctor, Edward Reynolds, who lived several blocks away. Joshua Merrill, a neighboring Methodist, often sent the nurses Sunday dinner. The sole clinical thermometer traveled from floor to floor in a basket on a pulley; surgery took place by gaslight in a cramped space on the top floor. Because there was no elevator, patients had to be carried up and down the four flights of stairs, usually by nurses. That practice was referred to in an anonymous note of the time as "difficult and dangerous" and an "improper and inhuman thing for nurses." The hospital did have soothing music, however. Nurses intoned morning and evening hymns, accompanied by an organ, and they often sang to patients individually.

In spite of its limitations, the hospital thrived, mainly due to the compassionate nursing care it provided. As surgeon Maurice Howe Richardson, who sent many patients to the new hospital, remarked, "The success of a surgeon's work is often dependent on the work of nurses. This has been of the highest order in this Hospital. The patients always refer to it in the warmest terms. They speak of the care as though they had felt thoroughly at home. No matter how good a hospital may be — and we have in Boston as good as any in the world — the home-like feeling is a great aid to recovery. Sick people have many complaints, and they find fault with all hospitals, but they complain as little of this as of any. They are so well pleased that they wish to go back again, when in need of treatment, which is the greatest of compliments."

A 1905 report likewise credited the hospital's early success to the devoted care and Christian atmosphere as well as to the skills of the surgeons. One young woman, whose life had been saved by a physician and by the untiring care of nurses, was reported to have undergone a spiritual awakening during her stay. It was observed, "She went from us a changed woman, the light of His presence in her face, the peace of Christ in her soul, carrying with her the atmosphere of helpfulness. She does not understand how anybody could remain long in the Hospital and not become a Christian." Another former patient wrote, "I shall never forget the loving, faithful care I received in your Hospital." And yet

First home of New England Deaconess Hospital, 691 Massachusetts Avenue, ca. 1896. Dedicated on February 5, 1896, the new hospital was described by one contemporary journalist as "a model of its kind." Housed in a five-story former residence, the small facility included a dining room, kitchen, laundry, fourteen patient beds, a medical floor, a surgical floor, and rooms for nurses. Early supporters lauded the hospital's efficient approach to providing care: ". . . a single nurse could care for a half-dozen patients, gathered into a hospital ward, who would, if scattered through their inconvenient and unsanitary homes, have required the whole time of a half-dozen nurses."

another, "This is the anniversary of my operation in your Hospital and I could not refrain from writing to those among whom some of my happiest days were spent."

BUILDING A STAFF AND FILLING BEDS

As superintendent, Mary Lunn oversaw all aspects of patient care. Abbie L. Punchard, who had been trained at Salem Hospital, became the hospital's first head nurse, but illness soon forced her to step down. Following another woman's short tenure, M. Elizabeth Booker, a graduate of Massachusetts General Hospital's nursing school, assumed the position of head nurse. "Miss Booker, a woman of strong character and professional skill," the brief 1940 history observed, "organized and systematized the little hospital and made it popular with both doctors and patients." The early hiring of these supervisory nurses to teach the deaconesses and oversee patient care indicated Lunn's belief in the advantages of professional training. It also presaged the future of the nursing school.

Although doctors provided lectures for nursing students, most of the training was bedside, under the supervision of the head nurse and superintendent. In 1898 the hospital graduated its first class of nurses, three in number and all deaconesses. The following year instruction was broadened and non-deaconesses were admitted. By 1904 training was increased from two to three years, including a probationary period and six months of nursing outside the hospital. This continuing expansion of the course of study was in keeping with national trends. Indeed, the school's very founding coincided with a great nationwide proliferation of nursing schools: in 1880, there were 15 programs in the United States; by 1900, that number had mushroomed to 432.

When non-deaconesses first began to outnumber deaconesses among the hospital's trainees is not known, though probably not many years after the program's establishment. Candidates for admission were still required to be Christians, however, although Catholics were excluded. Many of the young women who came to train were Methodists from small towns and cities across New England. And characteristic of such programs of the day, the school closely monitored the behavior, especially the moral conduct, of its students, and enforced strict discipline. Few students were married. Indeed, in 1898 a married probationer who desired to be a nursing student was admitted on the condition that her husband co-sign the contract with her.

In addition to the deaconesses and nursing trainees, the new hospital had an open medical staff, welcoming all physicians in good standing. Patients were permitted to have their own doctors, provided payment either was made in advance or was satisfactorily guaranteed. Non-paying patients were allowed their choice of doctors, whose services the hospital required to be given without charge. Like many facilities in these years, the Deaconess did not at the outset admit chronic, contagious, or convalescent cases, at least officially. In an early circular, however, the hospital quoted one of its physicians extolling the Deaconess's excellent work with chronic cases. The hospital's 1902 annual report noted that the average length of stay was 25 days; the longest time for any patient was 182 days.

The hospital's founding coincided with the increasing popularity of surgery as a desired mode of treatment for the middle and upper classes. Because of the new role hospitals were assuming, Boston did not have enough private beds to meet the growing demand, even though the city was home to a number of institutions. In addition to Massachusetts General, which had opened its doors in 1821, the city accommodated Boston City Hospital (1864), one of the country's first municipal hospitals; New England Hospital for Women and Children, founded in 1862 by women doctors for women patients; Children's Hospital, established by four physicians in 1869; Carney Hospital, a Roman Catholic institution which opened in South Boston, also in 1869; St. Margaret's, begun by members of an Anglican religious order in the 1880s; and Boston Baptist Hospital, which first accepted patients in 1894 and subsequently changed its name to New England Baptist Hospital.

Although questions arose internally about the uniform quality of the medical staff, from the outset the Deaconess attracted a number of leading practitioners as well as those beginning their medical practices, many of whom would achieve prominence later. Heading the list was Maurice Howe Richardson, a renowned surgeon at Massachusetts General, who became Moseley Professor of Surgery at Harvard. Frustrated by the paucity of private beds at Massachusetts General as well as by that hospital's policy, which prohibited doctors from collecting professional fees from patients, Richardson was frank in saying that he depended on his practice for his livelihood. He reported learning about the Deaconess by chance from his colleague, Edward Reynolds, and was soon one of the hospital's busiest practitioners and most loyal friends. "From that time to this I have been harassed by the fact that I could not get beds enough," Richardson commented for a Deaconess fund-raising circular in 1901. "There have been many times when I and my assistants could fill all the beds there, but it is so full that it is well-nigh impossible." Richardson's comments obviously indicate both a thriving surgical practice and a shortage of private hospital beds. In addition to being a highly regarded surgeon, Richardson was a warm individual, sometimes playing hymns and songs for patients and deaconesses alike. He also brought freshly caught fish to the nurses. "His eyes would twinkle when, after Miss Lunn had lectured him for fishing on Sunday, she would eat the fish!" a 1948 hospital history noted. Richardson's young assistant, Daniel Fiske Jones, who was fond of wearing a carnation in his lapel, was also remembered for his warmth and genuine concern for patients.

Another prominent member of the Deaconess staff was Fanny Berlin. A native of Russia who had joined the Revolutionary Party as a young woman, Berlin subsequently migrated to Switzerland and received her medical training at the University of Zurich. She arrived in Boston in the late 1870s and soon established herself as a pioneer woman surgeon and a staff member at New England Hospital for Women and Children. Berlin also developed a private practice, and that, it may be surmised, is why she joined the staff of the new Deaconess Hospital.

Among the hospital's young physicians was Joel E. Goldthwait, a thirty-year-old orthopedic surgeon who had held a minor staff position at Children's Hospital for three years. In 1922 Goldthwait would write the doctors' bible on posture. Another promising doctor was the young Elliott P. Joslin, who began to practice medicine in 1898. Born in Oxford, Massachusetts, in 1869, Joslin attended Yale College and Harvard Medical School, from which he graduated in 1895. He subsequently won a competitive appointment to the staff of Boston City Hospital, became an assistant in the Department of Physiological Chemistry at Harvard Medical School, and joined the staff of New England Deaconess Hospital.

CONSISTENT WITH WHAT WAS OCCURRING NATIONALLY, a large majority of the patients admitted to the Deaconess in the early years were surgical, not medical. In the year ending May 1900, for example, the hospital performed

135 operations, 57 of which it classified as major, 78 as minor. In 1902, there were 156 surgical patients and 29 medical. The hospital also trumpeted its low mortality rate — after four years, 658 patients had been treated but only 22 had died. Like most hospitals at that time, the preponderance of patients were women, most of them "at home," that is, not working women. The hospital initially performed some maternity work, but, for reasons unreported, abandoned the service by 1900.

The Deaconess boasted that in addition to attracting many patients from Massachusetts, it also drew from other New England states, from the Canadian maritime provinces, and from even more distant places. Likewise, though it treated many Methodists, the Deaconess also prided itself on its patients' religious diversity. "While we call ours a Methodist Hospital, and hope it may have all the Christian sweetness and good cheer which Methodism stands for," declared Willard T. Perrin for the Board of Managers in 1898, "its doors swing open with a cordial welcome to the suffering of every creed and race and social condition."

In keeping with both national and local trends, the Deaconess relied significantly on patients who paid their way in whole or in part. The 1900 report stated the hospital's intention to reserve half its beds for non-paying patients, "although the limitations are such in the present building that this plan cannot always be carried out." Indeed, not. In the hospital's first four years, 88 (13 percent) patients paid nothing, 191 (29 percent) paid something, and 379 (58 percent) paid full price. In other words, 100 more patients paid full price than were either wholly or partly charitable. Paying patients also generally paid their doctors' private fees. Thus, from the outset, the Deaconess was not strictly or even primarily a charity hospital, though it was one in part.

In these early days, the deaconesses and the nursing trainees made the hospital economically viable by working without salary. Paying patients effectively subsidized non-paying ones or those who paid part of their costs. The hospital, though administered by a lay committee, was dependent on doctors for filling its beds, especially paying beds, suggesting that applicants for admission had to be recommended by a doctor. "Physicians of recognized standing can bring patients and treat them as exclusively as in the patient's home," the hospital's superintendent noted in 1904.

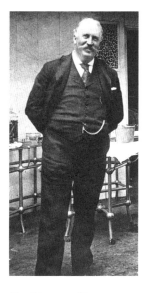

DR. MAURICE HOWE RICHARDSON, CA. 1900. *One of Deaconess Hospital's first doctors and most devoted friends, Richardson was regarded as one of the foremost surgeons of his time. A busy practitioner who consulted at a number of hospitals, Richardson would often traverse three states in one day visiting patients and performing surgery.*

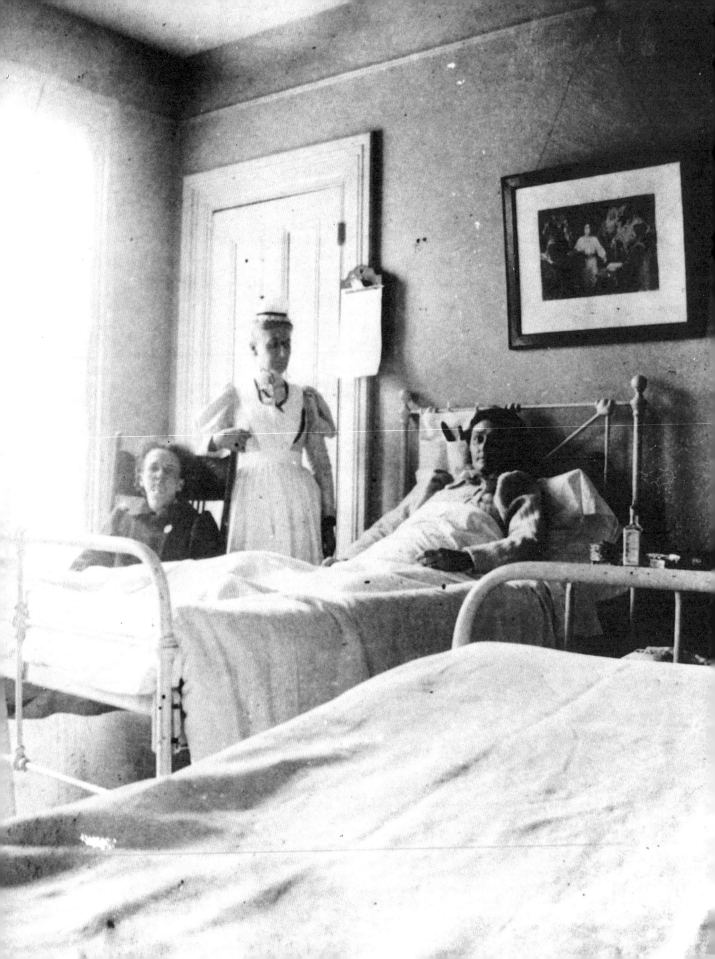

Thus, like many American hospitals, the New England Deaconess, from its earliest years, actually had multiple purposes and met multiple needs: it was both religious and secular, charitable and private in its orientation, fulfilling the Christian purposes of its Methodist founders while serving the professional, secular needs of doctors, primarily surgeons, who were keen to find beds and excellent nursing care for their private patients. As was true of many hospitals, the Deaconess was both a doctors' workshop *and* an independent, altruistic institution.

However complex, the formula worked. Indeed, the Deaconess was quickly filled to capacity and could not meet the demand. "The great need is lack of beds," observed Richardson. "A hospital of ten times the size could easily be kept full." Some of the best surgeons in Boston had become the hospital's "cordial friends," Willard Perrin wrote in 1898, "and are constantly urging the enlargement of our work. Where is the kind friend who will give us $20,000 at once and leave us as much or more in his will?" he wondered.

MOVING TO THE WOODS

The hospital's obvious success, the confidence of doctors that they could fill additional beds, and the inherent shortcomings of the original building soon combined to make a compelling case for a new site. Thus, in 1900, the New England Deaconess Association voted $26,500 for the purchase of a lot on the Riverway in the Longwood section of Boston with the idea of building a new fifty-bed Deaconess Hospital, at an anticipated cost of $100,000. It was Mary Lunn who recommended, indeed insisted on, this particular site, and it was she who was reportedly criticized for it. "You can't expect doctors to go to the woods to treat their patients," several early histories reported people saying. The Riverway was not quite as radical a choice as legend would have it, however. Downtown areas of Boston were crowded, and prime property was expensive. Inner Boston also had ample hospital service — Massachusetts General, Boston City, and Carney hospitals. Meanwhile, Boston's population was expanding westward, toward Longwood, Brookline, Jamaica Plain, Roxbury, and West Roxbury, all of which, with the exception of Brookline, became part of Boston.

HOLT ROOM, New England Deaconess Hospital, ca. 1897. Located on the medical floor, the Holt Room was one of the early hospital rooms dedicated as memorials to prominent Methodists. The hospital's compassionate care and homelike atmosphere were planned from the beginning, as an early advocate noted, "We do not want it [the hospital] to be merely an institution, but more of a Home."

The advent of electric streetcars made these attractive new suburbs easily accessible to downtown — the Deaconess's projected new home was only a thirteen-minute streetcar ride from Park Street. Historian Sam Bass Warner has written, "Boston in 1900 was very much a city divided. With the exception of the Back Bay, it was an inner city of work and low-income housing, and an outer city of middle- and upper-income residences."

Institutional Boston followed the movement of people. In 1903 Isabella Stewart Gardner opened her unique museum in the Fenway. New England Baptist Hospital, whose history paralleled that of the Deaconess in many respects, began in a single room in Roxbury in 1893, moved to a house in the Longwood area the following year, then to a mansion on Parker Hill Avenue in Roxbury to a site atop Mission Hill. In 1904, fifteen prominent doctors, including Maurice Howe Richardson, organized Corey Hill Hospital in Brookline, which offered private patients pleasant suburban surroundings and experienced nursing care.

What was to prove the most important westward movement of any Boston institution, however, was the construction of a consolidated new Harvard Medical School on the Francis Estate in the Longwood area. The school's faculty, which had endorsed the move in 1900, was enticed to the location partly by the prospect of a new hospital to be built on this site, provided for in the will of real estate investor Peter Bent Brigham. Unlike the new Johns Hopkins medical school in Baltimore, which had achieved dominance in medical education and research almost from its opening in 1893, Harvard did not have control of a hospital, a circumstance which Harvard's leaders hoped to ameliorate with the new location.

Whether Lunn chose the Riverway site *because* she knew that Harvard was planning to move nearby is not known. In its 1902 report, however, Deaconess Hospital turned Harvard's plans to its own fund-raising advantage: "The site for the new hospital is in Longwood, Boston, about three minutes walk from the site of the proposed new Medical School of Harvard College, which is the largest and best equipped institution of its kind in the world."

Since the hospital had no legitimate ties to Harvard at this point, the implied connection appears in retrospect to have been somewhat self-serving. Whether the result of clever choice or sheer serendipity, however, locating the Deaconess proximate to Harvard Medical School would in time turn out to be one of the most significant decisions in the hospital's history.

Although she was responsible for choosing the new site, Lunn did not see the new hospital materialize; she resigned as superintendent in April of 1901. Whether she left due to illness, because she took another superintendency in New York, or for some other reason, perhaps controversy over site selection, is not known. Hospital minutes only indicate that she turned down an offer of a year's vacation with a deaconess allowance of $250.

In September 1901, Adeliza A. Betts, a native of Nova Scotia, a deaconess, and a member of the first nursing class of 1898, was named acting superintendent. The next year, at forty-nine years of age, she became superintendent on a permanent basis and was also named director of nursing and the nursing school. Betts was cited in hospital histories for her total dedication and unselfishness, praised for giving her own bed to a patient when none other was available and at times sleeping on chairs in her office. It was reported that she prepared her students for their examinations by quizzing them as they "scrubbed the floors or the instruments in the operating room." Betts retired in 1923 and died in the nurses' residence in 1934. Her administration "demonstrated her kindly wisdom and her gentle gracious personality," noted the 1940 history. Unfortunately, not much more evidence than this has survived about Betts's personality or style, but it appears that she was an inspiring and effective leader. Certainly she was successful, for what Lunn had envisaged, Betts brought to fruition.

IN 1903 THE FOUNDATION FOR THE NEW BUILDING was begun and the cornerstone laid. Further progress was halted, however, until funds could be raised for the superstructure. Within three years the deaconesses' dedication as well as the hospital's success inspired donors to complete a $50,000 subscription. In April of 1907 the three-story, fifty-bed Deaconess Hospital was completed and occupied. Like the original brownstone hospital, the new building was actually only one wing of what had originally been planned, doubtless owing to lack of funds. The hospital flourished in its expanded quarters. Within five years, more than fifty doctors were caring for patients in the new building and would have referred even more had the hospital's capacity been greater. In 1916 alone, the Deaconess admitted 1,409 patients, which was about as many as the hospital had cared for during its entire first nine years.

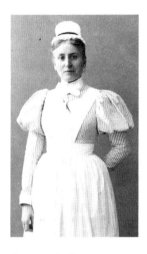

ADELIZA A. BETTS, CA. 1900. *The second superintendent of Deaconess Hospital, Betts was a graduate of the New England [Deaconess] Home and Training School and one of the first three graduates of the Nurses' Training School, Class of 1898. A native of Nova Scotia, Betts long wanted to become a nurse, but, due to family obligations, had to postpone the start of her career. Succeeding Mary Lunn as superintendent, Betts served Deaconess Hospital for more than twenty years and died in the nurses' residence in 1934 at age 81.*

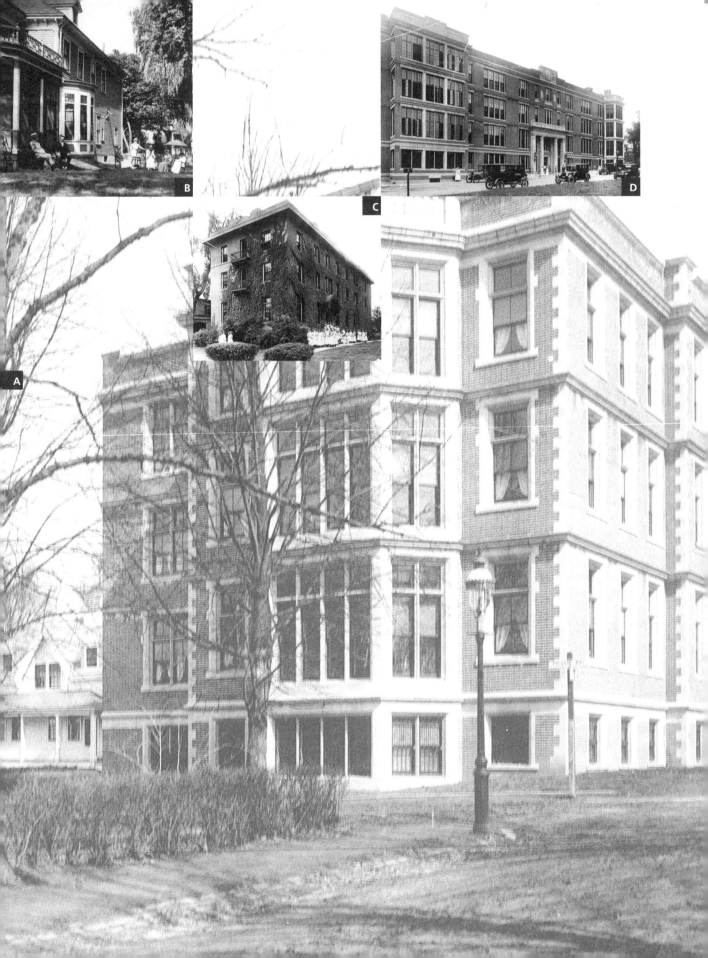

Four years after the hospital moved into its new building, the New England Deaconess Association struck out in a new direction when it opened a twenty-five-bed branch hospital in Concord, Massachusetts, called the Concord Deaconess Hospital. The facility was made possible by Charles Emerson, a nephew of Ralph Waldo Emerson and a Concord resident, who donated money and a hundred acres of land in gratitude for the excellent care his wife had received at Deaconess Hospital in Boston. The Concord Deaconess Hospital thrived at first, thanks in part to its busy obstetrical service and in part to the student nurses provided by Boston. In 1918 ninety-nine children were born in the Concord facility, whereas none was delivered at the Boston Deaconess. But by 1922, relations between the parent hospital and its branch were evidently strained and Concord began to run a large deficit, perhaps because Boston had stopped providing it with nurses. By 1924 the New England Deaconess Association had transferred control of the branch to a local board of managers. The Concord institution was later renamed and operates today as Emerson Hospital.

Expansion in Boston itself proceeded more smoothly. In 1913 Norman Wait Harris, a Methodist banker from Chicago, donated funds in his mother's memory for the construction of a new deaconess training building near the hospital. Named Harris Hall, the new facility became known as the Training School for Christian Service.

In 1913 the Deaconess Nurses' Training School began a long association with Simmons College, which provided science education for the hospital's nursing students. An academic affiliation was in keeping with ideas propounded by contemporary American nursing educators and reformers, such as Adelaide Nutting. Academic relationships upgraded the intellectual content of nursing education and slowly began to move training away from the exclusive control of hospitals. To provide its students with a well-rounded course of study, the school also aligned with other hospitals, such as Boston Lying-In in 1915 and Children's in 1920, which offered services the Deaconess lacked. In addition, nursing students had opportunities to work with the poor, either in their homes or in medical missions.

More changes and challenges lay ahead. In 1917, the Deaconess training school, that is, everything *but* nursing, began to merge with the

A DEACONESS HOSPITAL, 1907. *The hospital's second home at 175 Bellevue Street (renamed Pilgrim Road in 1912) in the Longwood section of Boston increased patient capacity from 14 to 50. Designed by Kendall Taylor & Stevens, Architects, of Boston, the December 1900 issue of the* New England Deaconess Journal *described the new facility as "a twentieth century hospital in every respect."*

B BRODBECK COTTAGE, CA. 1915. *Named for the first president of the New England Deaconess Association Board of Managers and housed in a building adjacent to the new hospital, Brodbeck was originally intended for use by both diabetic and nervous patients but soon became the center for Elliott P. Joslin's work on diabetes.*

C HARRIS HALL, CA. 1917. *Dedicated on September 24, 1913, as the new quarters of the Training School for Christian Service, the building later became home to generations of students of the New England Deaconess School of Nursing.*

D THE FOUR-STORY 1923 HOSPITAL ADDITION *increased patient beds to 175.*

Department of Religious Education at the Methodist-affiliated Boston University. The union culminated in 1922 when the executive committee of the Deaconess Association "with much regret, voted that the use of Harris Hall be withdrawn from the School of Religious Education and that it be used for the time being, at least, as a Home and Training School for Nurses." In 1922 the Deaconess nursing school had forty-three student nurses and thirteen probationers, but the committee looked forward to expanding enrollment. Five years later, in 1927, an addition to Harris Hall was built to provide accommodations for 170 or more students as well as supervisory personnel.

Despite this growing secularization, deaconesses continued to exert a strong influence over the training of nurses. Most important, their dedication to patient care established a standard and tradition that indelibly marked succeeding generations of nurses trained at the hospital. Adeliza Betts herself did not retire until 1923 and her successor as superintendent, Caroline A. Jackson, a graduate of the class of 1917, was also a deaconess. Nonetheless, young women were clearly increasingly interested in pursuing professional nursing, not a religious vocation, of which nursing was only one dimension.

As female employment in the economy increased alongside industrialization and urbanization, professional nursing provided large numbers of women with work and career opportunities. Hospital-trained nurses could serve as staff nurses or private-duty nurses in hospitals or they could work in physicians' offices and in public health positions. For a small number, who became head nurses, supervisors, and administrators, nursing provided additional upward mobility and professional opportunity. The feminization of the nursing profession had consequences, however, as recent historians of nursing have noted, for it helped assure nursing's subordination to medicine, which was dominated by men. One of the first rules that early student nurses learned was that the physician was always her director. The feminization of the profession also fostered the traditional role of women as nurturing caretakers in both their social and professional lives.

IN THE DEACONESS ASSOCIATION'S 1915 REPORT, President Willard Perrin hailed the hospital's expanding fortunes — with gross capital in property and funds of $497,000 — and plainly told his readers exactly who deserved the credit: "The success of the work is due to the deaconesses — due to their service of sacrifice which appeals to people and brings in the money — due to their serving without salary, which makes it possible to conduct the work at less expense." He further alluded to a prevailing suspicion that certain people of ample means, including strong churches and well-paid ministers, were taking advantage of the situation to get service for themselves at reduced rates, thus preventing the deaconesses from serving the needs of the poor. "Such conduct is contemptible, indeed," he concluded.

Perrin went on to describe the Association's plight. "We cannot justly put off the completion of the Hospital in Boston. But the greatest need now as ever, is more deaconesses. What can be done to bring the young women of Methodism the vision of their duty and privilege?" Perrin beseeched. It can be inferred from Perrin's plea that young women were not coming forward in droves to become deaconesses; more often, young women simply wanted to become nurses.

THE GROWTH OF MEDICAL SPECIALTIES

At the end of the nineteenth century, specialization became an important phenomenon within medicine. Specialties initially developed according to age and gender — men, women, and children; by disease, such as gout, mental disorders, and consumption; and along anatomical and physiological divisions, such as the nervous, digestive, and respiratory systems. By 1915, there were an estimated thirty-four medical specialties. While general practice languished in the relatively barren economic soil of the countryside, specialization grew in the fertile soil of cities. According to historian Stanley Joel Reiser, by 1929, in cities with populations over 100,000, 35 percent of doctors were full-time specialists.

Not surprisingly, specialists became an important component of New England Deaconess Hospital. Elliott Joslin had started out as a general practitioner with a particular concentration on intestinal problems. But following an internship at Massachusetts General Hospital and several trips to leading laboratories in Germany and Austria, he developed an interest in diabetes. Joslin then traveled to Strasbourg to study under Bernard Naunyn, the world's leading specialist in that disease. When Joslin opened his office in his father's house on Beacon Street in Boston in 1898, he gradually narrowed the focus of his practice to diabetes, a

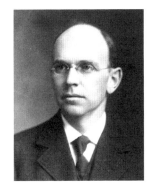

DR. ELLIOTT P. JOSLIN, CA. 1920. *Associated with Deaconess Hospital from 1898, Joslin became one of the world's leading authorities on the care and treatment of diabetics. A pioneer in teaching diabetic patients and their families the proper management of the disease, Joslin was also known for his kindliness and human touch.*

chronic, devastating, and often fatal disease. In 1908 Joslin began to conduct research on a series of diabetic cases.

Diet (actually undernutrition nearly to starvation) was then the only known way to treat diabetes. "Joslin tended to be optimistic about the therapy," historian Michael Bliss has written. "He was almost certainly over-optimistic, possibly deliberately so to bolster his patients' morale and his own. It was hard to keep up your spirits to face each day of urging sick people to keep starving. Because he tempered his own rock-hard puritanism with warmth and charm and a sense of hope, Joslin may have had more success with his patients than the forbidding Dr. [Frederick] Allen [of Morristown, New Jersey, one of America's other leading diabetologists]." Joslin "was particularly popular with children," Bliss has noted, "some of whom were brought to him because no one else would treat them."

Joslin's work included studying patients' metabolism following ingestion of carefully selected and measured foods. He became associated with Francis G. Benedict, the director of the Carnegie Nutrition Laboratory, which was located in the Longwood area between Harvard Medical School and Deaconess Hospital. There, and at the Deaconess itself, Joslin, both on his own and collaboratively, was able to carry out important metabolic research and to publish several classic works on the science and treatment of diabetes.

In November 1915, under Joslin's influence and guidance, the Deaconess opened the William Nast Brodbeck Cottage adjacent to the hospital. The building, which had belonged to the first president of the Board of Managers and was named in his honor, expanded the capacity of the hospital from fifty to seventy beds and was dedicated to the care of "diabetic and nervous patients," but it was diabetic patients who quickly predominated. Filled to capacity from the beginning, Brodbeck soon had a long waiting list; five additional beds were shoehorned in. Most Brodbeck patients were of modest circumstances, but were not charity cases; there were only two private rooms, and most patients shared a room with one, two, or three others.

A visionary teacher as well as an outstanding clinician, Joslin developed Brodbeck into a kind of school. One of his central purposes was to instruct patients in how to care for themselves after they left the hospital. Nurses were given specialized training in diabetic treatment, enabling them to assist patients in their home communities and to work as diabetes specialists in other hospitals. Moreover, physicians, first from around the United States and, by 1919, from around the world, came to Brodbeck to learn about the latest treatment methods.

Brodbeck also housed clinical research. Through the courtesy of the Carnegie Nutrition Laboratory, "a respiratory apparatus" was installed in the building to perform scientific observations. Carnegie also supplied a technician, Marion L. Baker, to run a chemical laboratory. "We know of but two institutions in the country where highly specialized work of this type is attempted," the Deaconess Association's 1916 annual report proudly asserted. Joslin himself noted in the 1922 report how unusual it was for scientific work of this type to be carried out in a private hospital. Usually, it was conducted "only in medical schools or in public hospitals with free patients," he remarked. "All of the investigations thus far carried on with diabetic patients at the Deaconess Hospital have been with private patients, not charity patients. Their cooperation has contributed to its success."

The great breakthrough in the treatment of diabetes was made by two Canadians at the University of Toronto in the summer of 1921. Working in the laboratory of Professor J. J. R. Macleod, Frederick G. Banting and Charles H. Best, a doctor and chemistry student respectively, succeeded in bringing a diabetic dog out of coma through the use of insulin, a pancreatic extract. Later that year Joslin attended the famous session of the American Physiological Society at Yale University where Macleod, Banting, and Best reported their findings. Many of the experts present, including Joslin, were wary. George H. A. Clowes, research director of Eli Lilly and Company, an Indiana-based pharmaceutical manufacturer, thought the evidence convincing and asked the Canadians whether his company could collaborate with them in preparing the extract commercially. An arrangement was made.

By the summer of 1922, Eli Lilly's "Iletin" was being made available for clinical trials by selected physicians. Joslin himself received his first supply on August 6 and was so excited about the treatment's potential that he could not sleep that night. Indeed, the next day he was reportedly too nervous to give the first injection himself, so it was administered by his assistant physician, Howard F. Root. The diabetic recipient was a forty-two-year-old former nurse, Elizabeth Mudge, who had almost starved to death under a strict dietary regimen. Mudge

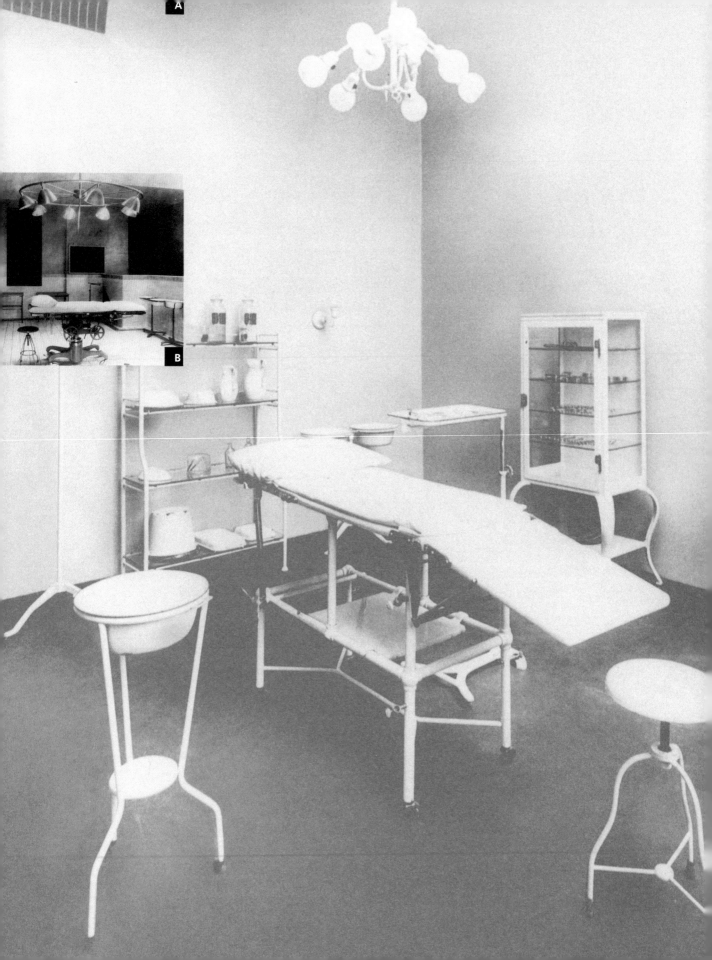

had grown so weak that she could not move. Within ten days of starting insulin treatment, she was carrying trays for other patients. Within six weeks, she was walking four miles a day. And with insulin therapy and continued adherence to diet, Mudge lived another twenty-five years.

During the remainder of 1922, other patients received treatment under Joslin. "The sole criterion of the selection of patients to have this remedy, which until 1923 could not be bought," Joslin reported, "has been severity of the disease and faithfulness to dietetic rules. What a privilege it has been to watch the development of this epoch-making discovery!" Indeed, it was a medical miracle, but Joslin realized that diabetes was still not cured by insulin, that diet remained terribly important in the management of the disease. "With boundless energy, a deep sense of mission, and considerable public relations skill," Michael Bliss writes, "Joslin continued to expand his facilities and his staff in Boston, becoming the 'master clinician' of diabetes." In 1925 Harvard promoted Joslin to clinical professor of medicine.

ROENTGENOLOGY WAS ANOTHER SPECIALTY that found a home at the Deaconess. In late 1895, Wilhelm Roentgen, a professor of physics at the University of Würzburg in Bavaria, first reported on his discovery of new rays which he called X rays because of their unknown composition. Their ability to see through solid objects quickly captured the popular imagination and the obvious potential to see inside the body understandably captivated physicians as well. Walter B. Cannon, while still in medical school at Harvard in 1896, began to investigate the digestive tract with X rays through the use of ingested bismuth. By 1901, approximately 8,000 patients had been X-rayed at Massachusetts General Hospital.

In 1916 the Deaconess acquired its first X-ray machine, which was installed in a ground-floor room. In addition to diagnostic applications, the equipment was sometimes used for treatment, especially in goiter cases. The modality was soon added to the hospital's diagnostic and treatment armamentarium. More than 700 plates were made at the Deaconess in 1918; 10 years later, 3,000 X rays were processed.

At the time the hospital acquired its first X-ray machine, it also appointed Lawrie B. Morrison as the first staff roentgenologist, as radiologists were then called. A native of Vermont and a graduate of the University of Vermont Medical School, Morrison had a scientific bent

A DEACONESS HOSPITAL OPERATING ROOM, 1907. *The hospital's new surgical facility was an improvement over the single surgical bed and gas lamps of the original site. Dedicated to fostering both compassionate patient care and scientific achievement, the planners of the new building incorporated the very latest ideas in construction and equipment to ensure a "scientifically up to date" facility.*

B DEACONESS HOSPITAL OPERATING ROOM, 1923. *The hospital's new four-story addition expanded the surgical facilities and permitted the handling of additional procedures that followed with increased patient capacity. The opening of a "Pathological Laboratory" next to the operating rooms facilitated microscopic examination of tissue removed during surgery.*

and did pioneering research at the Deaconess, including work on vascular calcification, especially in diabetics. Tragically, like many early radiologists, he was overexposed to radiation and developed cancer in his fingers and hands. Despite progressive amputations, Morrison continued to attend patients and conduct research courageously almost until his death in 1933.

The arrival of Frank H. Lahey in 1914 had also strengthened the hospital's reputation as a specialty institution. Born in Haverhill, Massachusetts, in 1880, Lahey was the son of an Irish mother and a successful contractor whose father had been an immigrant Irish laborer. A graduate of Harvard Medical School, Lahey trained as a surgeon at Boston City Hospital and became resident surgeon at the Haymarket Relief Station, a branch of City Hospital. Just as Joslin developed diabetes as a specialty at the Deaconess, Lahey focused on the surgical treatment of goiter cases and thyroid conditions, though he never confined himself strictly to these areas and always regarded himself as a general surgeon. By the end of 1919, Lahey had cared for 228 goiter and thyroid cases at the Deaconess and the hospital's annual report included a section on "The Goitre Clinic," which immediately followed that on "The Diabetic Clinic."

Under Lahey's leadership, in 1919 the hospital set aside a small room for clinical research and equipped it with a Benedict portable respirometer for the estimation of basal metabolism. By the end of 1920, 450 metabolism examinations had been carried out under the direction of Sara M. Jordan, Lahey's young assistant. The tests were enormously helpful diagnostically as well as in determining the timing and extent of any operation, and Lahey was the first Boston surgeon to make use of these findings. In 1920 he performed 168 thyroid operations with only three deaths, a significant achievement in an area that had formerly carried grave risk. Lahey attributed the low mortality rate (1.8 percent) to three factors: "(1) that we have in this Hospital all the facilities for the proper study of these cases; (2) that we have a special group for the study and care of these cases; (3) because of our extensive and increasing experience with this particular type of disease."

Lahey's remarkable success brought a flood of desperate patients to his door. By 1922, "The Thyroid Clinic," as it was now called, had performed 450 operations on patients who came from throughout the northeastern United States and eastern Canada. Business was so brisk that not all cases could even be accommodated at the Deaconess. Of the 376 thyroid operations conducted there, only one death occurred. Lahey did not feel that such a low mortality rate (0.3 percent) could be sustained, however, and was prepared to sacrifice that impressive statistic to try to save desperately ill patients.

A number of thyroid patients also had cardiac problems. In fact, some patients who arrived at the clinic died of heart failure within hours. For the majority, however, once they had been properly prepared and medicated, Lahey was able to operate successfully. Few contemporary surgeons would have even attempted to do what Lahey achieved virtually as a matter of routine. With the clinic's cardiac-related work expanding rapidly, the hospital installed its first electrocardiograph in 1922.

The specialized research and care provided by both Lahey and Joslin and their colleagues began to focus a national spotlight on New England Deaconess Hospital. During the meeting of the American College of Surgeons in Boston in 1922, for example, clinics on diabetes and thyroid disease were held at the hospital and its facilities. "These Clinics were attended daily by from one hundred to two hundred and fifty surgeons from all States in the Union, from Mexico, Cuba and South America," noted Lahey, who was already proving to be both a brilliant promoter and organizer as well as a consummate surgeon.

WAR AND RECOVERY

During World War I, the hospital temporarily lost the services of both Lahey and Joslin as well as a number of other doctors and nurses. And those who stayed behind had to double their efforts, for the hospital remained almost as busy as before. In the patriotic atmosphere immediately preceding American entry into the war in 1917, the hospital had established a preparedness committee, chaired by William T. Rich, a member of the Board of Managers. One of its members was Daniel Fiske Jones, who had returned from six months as a battlefield surgeon in France.

The committee concluded that the most practical thing the hospital could do was to build a temporary facility for the care of wounded soldiers. William Rich himself enthusiastically advanced the necessary funds. The Willard T. Perrin Ward, named for the hospital's

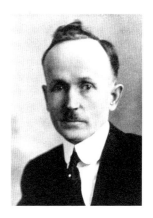

DR. LAWRIE B. MORRISON, CA. 1927. *Founder of the Deaconess Department of Radiology, Morrison was a trained pathologist and medical professor before he moved to Boston to study radiology at Massachusetts General Hospital. Morrison also established radiology departments at the University of Vermont and at New England Baptist, Faulkner, Robert Breck Brigham, and Corey Hill hospitals. Like others who suffered from X-ray exposure, Morrison underwent several amputations but continued to work until November 1932. He died in January of 1933.*

longtime president, rose on a vacant lot across from the hospital in the spring and summer of 1917. Though a simple frame structure, it attracted attention as the first war hospital in Boston. Indeed, 500 people inspected it on the day it opened. Doctors, it should be noted, patriotically donated their services. The contribution of the Deaconess to the war effort was modest compared to larger Boston medical institutions. Boston City, Massachusetts General, and Harvard Medical School each set up and ran base hospitals in Europe. Many of the Deaconess-affiliated doctors and nurses who went to war may have served at one of these facilities.

One hundred fifty enlisted men received care in the Perrin Ward in 1918, not only for war injuries but for influenza. Indeed, the flu devastated the country in 1918 and 1919, killing half a million Americans; worldwide, it was estimated to have caused twenty-two million deaths. By the end of October 1918, 17,000 men at Fort Devens, thirty miles west of Boston, had the flu and close to 800 had died. But thanks primarily to superb nursing care, only one flu victim died in the Perrin Ward. During the epidemic, Brodbeck Cottage was turned over to the state board of health for treatment of physicians and nurses who had come from out of state and had themselves contracted the flu. In July 1919, the Perrin Ward was dismantled and moved to Haverhill where it was used as a camp dormitory at the Deaconess Home that had been opened there.

AFTER THE WAR, Deaconess Hospital returned to its normal routine, that is, it became busier than ever. In 1919, 1,530 patients were admitted; in 1920, 1,625; and in 1922, 1,888. Surgical cases still predominated — 1,200 operations were performed in 1922, for example, 692 major and 508 minor. But clearly the work of Joslin and his assistants on diabetics was also placing ever greater demand on hospital capacity — in 1922 there were 782 medical admissions, a much higher proportion than in the hospital's early days.

The trend toward private cases was equally clear. In 1919 there were only 93 (6 percent) non-paying patients out of the 1,530, as compared to 13 percent in the Deaconess's first four years. By 1922, both the number of non-paying patients, 88, and the proportion had shrunk further. That year the hospital also recorded 73 part-pay patients and listed the value of its free work as more than $7,900. This trend at the Deaconess was, it should be noted, in keeping with what was happening nationally. "If we could visualize the . . .

divisions of the social strata as cream, milk, . . . and water, we could designate the private patient as the 'cream,' the semi-private patient as the 'milk,' and the pauper or indigent patient as the 'water,'" an administrator at another institution explained. Hospitals, like the doctors who worked in them, wanted a good dollop of the cream.

Rising admissions, the popularity of its specialized clinics, and the confidence of its doctors argued for hospital expansion, that is, fulfillment of the trustees' original plans. Consequently, in 1922 construction began on a major addition to the 1907 building. The new wing would more than double the size of the hospital, adding 125 beds upon completion in 1923. The expansion also resulted in relocating the hospital's main entrance from Pilgrim Road to Deaconess Road, where patients entered through an attractive vestibule and main hall leading to administrative offices, whose very existence suggested the growing size and complexity of the hospital organization.

The slope of the land allowed the new structure to gain a floor on the 1907 building, with four levels instead of three. The entire fourth floor was devoted to surgery and a large new operating room was constructed where the new joined the old. A four-room X-ray department and a medical laboratory were installed in the basement. The new building included such modern amenities as a nurse call system and two push-button elevators, one for passengers, the other for food and supplies. A special system provided ice-cold drinking water to each floor, eliminating the need for nurses to retrieve ice. The upper floors of the new structure had rear balconies where bedding and mattresses could be aired out discreetly. The balconies also were designed to allow patients in wheelchairs to relax without being exposed to the elements. The roof similarly had a sun room and a promenade for convalescent patients. A separate section for diabetic patients included an assembly hall for instruction and a dining room.

The attention to patients' comfort and convenience reflected a growing trend in the 1920s when American hospitals were becoming increasingly consumer- or market-driven. The most obvious manifestation of this development was the movement away from wards and toward private and semi-private rooms. Large hospitals were sometimes compared to multiclass hotels, trains, or ships, which offered different

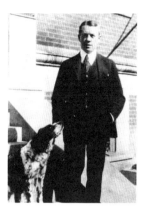

DR. FRANK H. LAHEY (AND "DIXIE"), CA. 1920. *A talented surgeon, teacher, and administrator, Lahey was a pioneer in the creation of multispecialty group medical practice and headed the nation's third-largest multi-specialist clinic. Affiliated with the Deaconess beginning in 1914, Lahey was an important and influential hospital presence for nearly four decades. Hunting dogs were one of Lahey's great interests; several he personally trained won national championships in the amateur class.*

accommodations at different prices. Adapting to this trend, the Deaconess offered private rooms, semi-private rooms, and small, medium-sized, and large wards.

Standardization and certification of hospitals also reflected the consumer environment of the 1920s. Certification assured consumers that a hospital met certain objective standards. The American College of Surgeons (ACS) began inspecting hospitals in 1918. In the 1920s, certification became tantamount to the "Good Housekeeping Seal of Approval," another voluntary program developed in that decade. Perhaps the most valuable contribution of the ACS was promoting the importance of pathology findings to surgery.

The Deaconess 1922 report indicated that "in order to meet the standardization requirements of the American College of Physicians and Surgeons [sic] a Permanent Medical and Surgical Staff has been organized and entered upon its duties on January 1, 1923." To meet the new requirements, the hospital also had to keep complete case records. The ACS favored permanent staffs, which gave doctors a mechanism both for exercising control over hospitals and for self-policing and quality assurance. Permanent staff organizations could, of course, be used for either good or ill — to exclude doctors because they were unqualified or unprofessional or on the basis of their race, religion, gender, or beliefs.

The first permanent hospital staff consisted of two surgeons, Jones and Lahey, and two physicians, Joslin and F. Gorham Brigham. In addition, there were four assistant physicians and surgeons, seven consultants listed by specialty (neurology, laryngology, roentgenology, ophthalmology, and dermatology), and forty-three associate members. Many of the hospital's staff members normally maintained other hospital affiliations, including Massachusetts General and Boston City. For several of the Deaconess's most distinguished doctors, however, the hospital was in fact a refuge from academic institutions. It was a place where they were free of teaching responsibilities and where their private patients could receive excellent care and not be poked and probed by medical students and interns. In contrast to the policy at some hospitals, moreover, the Deaconess did not limit or control doctors' fees.

The four members of the permanent staff became stars around whom some of the younger doctors orbited. Brigham, who had been one of Joslin's first two assistants (though there was no love lost between the two men), had set up his own private practice in Boston's Back Bay.

He also established the diabetes clinic at Massachusetts General. A big, vital man, Brigham had been captain of the Colgate University football and basketball teams. Bright, opinionated, and driven, Brigham dictated extensive notes about each patient and subsequently wrote his patients detailed letters describing his findings. So successful was he that other area physicians began to emulate his correspondence practices.

Brigham developed a huge private practice — when he retired he had files on approximately 16,000 patients. He employed an assistant physician primarily to take case histories and two stenographers and a secretary to take dictation and type. Although his patients included some ordinary folk, a significant number were well-to-do, referred to in those days as "silk-stocking" or "nice patients." They came from throughout New England and many adored him. Probably by the mid-1920s, Brigham was using the Deaconess for all or most of his hospitalizations and had become one of its dominant figures. It has been said that he would sweep into a patient's room, snip a flower from a bouquet, insert it in his lapel and announce that "the great Dr. Brigham" had arrived. "He's a bulwark, isn't he?" commented a typically admiring patient.

Lahey, by contrast, at 5 ft. 6 in., was short of stature, though certainly not self-confidence. Trim, erect, and immaculately groomed, Lahey was a creative, precise, and demanding surgeon. His vigor was infectious and he was a perfectionist. He was also hard-driving, dynamic, and charismatic, and he had a dream — the creation of a multispecialist group practice. Lahey was not the first person with such a vision. The Mayo brothers, Charles and William, established their clinic in Rochester, Minnesota, in 1914, and it soon became world famous. Military hospitals during World War I had also underscored the clinical advantages of multispecialist cooperation, to Lahey among others.

The medical profession itself was wary of group practice, however, alternately fearing that it would either commercialize practice or lead to socialized medicine. Lahey, however, was undeterred. In 1922, he persuaded gastroenterologist Sara Jordan, anesthesiologist Lincoln F. Sise, and fellow surgeon Howard M. Clute to join him in a group setting, which became known as the Lahey Clinic. Initially the practice operated out of an apartment on Beacon Street that Lahey and his wife had previously occupied.

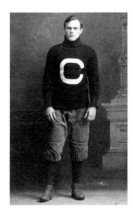

DR. F. GORHAM BRIGHAM, CA. 1904. *One of the hospital's first permanent staff members, Brigham's affiliation began in 1913 and continued for more than four decades until his retirement in 1955. Brigham was one of Joslin's early assistants and went on to found the diabetes clinic at Massachusetts General Hospital. In his college days at Colgate University, he served as captain of the varsity basketball and football squads.*

The members of Lahey's group became affiliated with the Deaconess as well as with New England Baptist Hospital, dividing their hospitalized patients between the two institutions. In 1923 Lahey was named to an unprecedented joint chair at Harvard and Tufts, but he resigned a year later to devote himself totally to his private group. Within two years of its founding, Lahey's "dream" became the third-largest clinic in the United States.

The other hospital staff surgeon, Daniel Fiske Jones, had served as Maurice Howe Richardson's assistant and then succeeded him. A leading surgeon and teacher at Massachusetts General, Jones followed Richardson's precedent by bringing along his associate, Leland S. McKittrick, who was listed as an "assistant surgeon" in 1923. Jones and McKittrick concentrated their private patients at the Deaconess and did perhaps half their work there. They were outstanding general surgeons, but were particularly involved in diabetic surgery, peripheral vascular disease, amputation, and cancer. Given several of their special interests, they naturally received many referrals from Joslin and his colleagues.

Joslin, the fourth member of the quadrumvirate, was a consummate New England Yankee, frugal by nature, recalled one of his associates, a man who would "squeeze a nickel until it screamed." He was a kind of medical priest for whom medicine was a high calling, not a path to wealth or to a life of ease. Any money saved should, in Joslin's view, be used to decrease costs to patients or to support research. He could seem austere and eccentric, but he actually had great warmth and sensitivity. Occasionally he displayed a wry sense of humor. When he was asked by a patient whether the use of a little alcohol now and then was permitted, Joslin replied, "absolutely not until you are over eighty."

Joslin had remarkable recall of patients and their conditions and he would call them to task if they did not take proper care of themselves, even if he just happened to see them in passing. An excellent organizer, Joslin had a knack for picking able subordinates and leaving them alone to do their jobs. He believed in a team approach to patient care, with various specialties and nursing each contributing its part. Joslin was also ahead of his time in his utilization of nurses to teach patients. His goal was to see the life span of diabetics exceed the norm. Like Lahey, Joslin was a visionary.

CANCER CARE, TREATMENT, AND RESEARCH

Five years after the completion of the new hospital wing, yet another structure rose in the growing Deaconess medical "complex." In April of 1927, adjacent to Deaconess Hospital, a handsome brick and concrete building opened its doors. Palmer Memorial Hospital, established under the auspices of the New England Deaconess Association, was dedicated to the care and treatment of cancer patients and other "incurables." The opening of the new building was marked by a week of festivities, including a round of speeches, meetings, and ceremonies attended by more than 2,500 visitors. Palmer Hospital cost over $750,000 to build, had seventy-five beds in private rooms and wards, a sun room on every floor, and a large solarium and library on the roof. The new hospital featured three operating rooms on the fourth floor and a small laboratory where a pathologist could prepare a frozen section of tissue and report quickly to a surgeon. "The lobby strikes the note of the building," wrote a contemporary chronicler. "It is the first indication of the pleasant atmosphere which includes everything for the patient's comfort, even the radio headset for every bed. . . . The entrance lobby . . . is so constructed that the patient who enters finds his or her spirits lifted at once. For the lobby is more like a cheerful hotel or a club than a hospital."

Palmer Hospital's history can be traced to 1919 when Jennie C. Palmer, a Methodist woman from Boston, was suffering from terminal cancer. At the time, relatively few hospitals in Boston would accept dying cancer patients. Even the Deaconess did not ordinarily admit incurable patients for more than three weeks. Before she died at the House of the Good Samaritan, a Catholic institution located near the Deaconess, Mrs. Palmer urged that a Protestant hospital be created to care for incurables. Her husband, William Lincoln Palmer, promised that he would do everything in his power to make her wish a reality. After she died, her plea became his crusade. Though not rich, Palmer had long been prominent in Methodism, knew many of its leaders, and was a tireless letter-writer and pamphleteer. Palmer's appeals fell on receptive ears at the New England Deaconess Association. Fortuitously, in 1920 the Association was given title to an attractive, rambling frame structure, the Cullis Consumptive Home on Blue Hill Avenue in Roxbury. Renamed Palmer

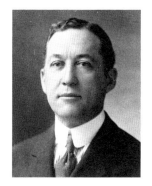

DR. DANIEL FISKE JONES, CA. 1910. *Jones became associated with the hospital early in his career while serving as an assistant to Maurice Howe Richardson. In 1923 he was appointed one of the first four permanent members of the hospital staff (along with surgeon Frank Lahey and physicians Gorham Brigham and Elliott Joslin). In 1927 Jones became surgeon-in-chief of the new Palmer Memorial Hospital. His many professional accomplishments included serving as president of the American Association of Surgeons.*

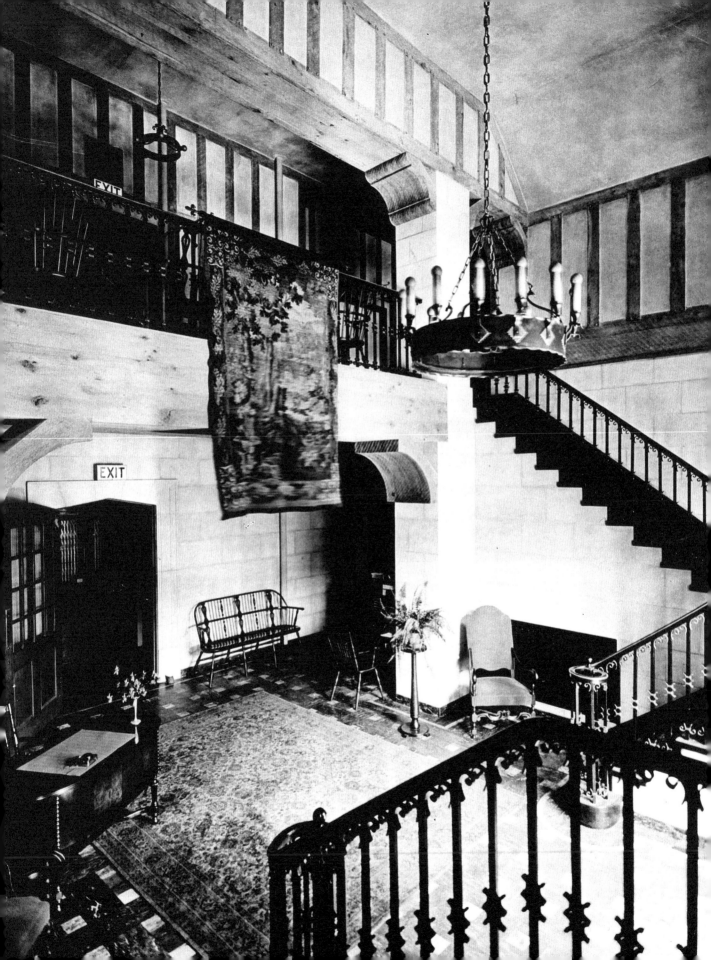

Memorial Hospital, it offered accommodations for thirty-nine incurable patients, primarily cancer sufferers. Serving as superintendent was Sadie A. Hagen, a Methodist deaconess, and its head nurse was Annie Raynes, also a deaconess and an early graduate of the Deaconess nursing school. The hospital gave sympathetic care to terminally ill patients, but it could not provide much in the way of treatment.

The exact details of the new Palmer Hospital's financing are unclear, though a confidential report of 1940 indicated that two large anonymous gifts, one for $125,000 and another for $250,000, would have accounted for about half its cost. Presumably the rest was financed by a mortgage. In the context of the booming economy of the 1920s, the entrepreneurial bent of its trustees, and previous successes with hospital expansion, the Association's optimism about its ability to retire debt would have been perfectly understandable. Indeed, these were promising years for American hospitals in general. Thanks to rising demand for beds, hospitals had a growing capacity to pay off capital costs simply by charging patients more. The last half of the 1920s brought a hospital construction boom in the United States that would not be matched again until the 1950s.

The new Palmer Hospital aimed to *treat* cancer patients through radiation and surgery, not merely to attend to them in their dying days. The hospital also sought to become part of an established cooperative endeavor, the Harvard Cancer Commission, to study cancer and improve its treatment. That commission was headed by Robert Greenough of Harvard Medical School and the nearby Huntington Memorial Hospital, which also specialized in cancer. "We now have here the best organized attack on the [cancer] problem that any American community has ever known," declared Greenough at the new Palmer Hospital's opening, "and to that attack the organization and personnel of the Palmer Memorial brings valuable and much needed assistance." In an early venture in cooperation and collaboration, the Palmer's radium was stored in a vault at Huntington Memorial and radon gas, derived from radium and used for certain cancer treatments, was brought as needed.

Palmer Hospital's first surgeon-in-chief was Daniel Fiske Jones, while Joslin was named chief physician. Appointed staff pathologist was a young physician, Shields Warren, who later cited Joslin and Lahey in his

FOYER OF PALMER MEMORIAL HOSPITAL, CA. 1927. *At the hospital's opening in April of 1927, a journalist detailed the Palmer's resplendent facility: "The lobby is an adaptation in antique natural oak, by heavy beams and paneling, so combined with soft gray stone as to reproduce an English baronial interior. A tapestry and tinted lamps add to the effect." The* Boston Medical and Surgical Journal *of April 28, 1927, hailed the Palmer as ". . . the largest institution in New England devoted to the care and treatment of the cancer patient. . . . It is not merely to be a refuge for the chronic sick, but it is to wage an aggressive campaign, armed with the best weapons known to medical science, against chronic disease, and particularly cancer."*

decision to join the Deaconess rather than accept more prestigious offers, including one from Massachusetts General. A graduate of Boston University and Harvard Medical School, Warren, a promising twenty-nine-year-old scientist, had trained in pathology under the eminent F. B. (Frank) Mallory at Boston City Hospital. "One of my men, Shields Warren, who received an appointment at the Harvard Medical School in pathology under the auspices of the Rockefeller Foundation, has just been appointed pathologist to the Deaconess Hospitals [sic] at a salary of $5000 to start with and a $500 increase yearly for ten years, some going for a man 2½ years out of the medical school," Mallory wrote a fellow pathologist in Kentucky. Warren thus became the first doctor to be employed directly by the Deaconess.

Warren had acquired from Mallory and from Francis Peabody at Boston City Hospital a keen interest in patients, which was somewhat unusual for a pathologist. He was fascinated by scientific research, but he shared with the Deaconess staff a belief in the importance of providing patients with the best care. Another attraction of the Deaconess was that it gave Warren the opportunity to set up a pathology laboratory from scratch. Before his arrival, much of the hospital's pathology work had been carried out independently. (There had been a chemical laboratory on site, however, directed by Hazel Hunt.) Six technicians performed routine work and two more conducted diabetes research. Joslin, Lahey, and McKittrick were among those who had pushed for the establishment of a pathology department and who subsequently selected Warren as the best person for the job.

In 1928, a year after Warren's arrival, he was named director of combined laboratories — chemical, pathology, metabolic, and electrocardiographic — with a staff that totaled fifteen. The pathology staff included five technicians and secretaries, a research assistant, *and* a resident, apparently the Deaconess's first. The hospital began to charge a flat rate of $5 to all ward patients and $7.50 to private room patients, which covered most laboratory tests regardless of length of stay.

Warren established a cohesive department to cover all clinical and anatomic pathology services, the first unified department of pathology in Boston, according to Merle A. Legg, a later chief of Deaconess pathology. A talented scientist, Warren quickly initiated research on the pathology of diabetes, made possible by Joslin's routine autopsies on deceased diabetics. Just three years after his arrival at the hospital, Warren published an important book on diabetes mellitus. He also soon became engaged in research on cancer of the thyroid, which was facilitated by the large volume of thyroid surgery performed by Lahey and his team. The resultant classification of thyroid tumors by Warren and Lahey became the standard in the field for many years.

Coincidentally, and unlike many Deaconess-affiliated doctors, Warren was a Methodist. Warren's grandfather was a Methodist minister who became the first president of Boston University. Warren's father was a faculty dean at Boston University, and he, himself, later served as a trustee and chairman of the board there. Yet when Warren was interviewed years later about why he chose to accept the Deaconess offer in 1927, he did not even mention its Methodist affiliation. It was presumably irrelevant to his decision, just like his Boston University link. After attending Harvard Medical School, Warren became an instructor there in 1925 and an assistant professor in 1936. A number of other Deaconess doctors, it should be added, were also members of Harvard's clinical faculty.

AT THE END OF 1927, chief surgeon Jones reported, "The most noteworthy and gratifying accomplishments of the year have been those patients who have been sent home with their disease [cancer] arrested. By having patients enter the Hospital for such treatment as is necessary, and then following them in the Out Patient Department, it is possible to make the beds of the Hospital far more useful in serving the community." Of the 997 patients admitted in 1928, 821 were discharged "improved." Unfortunately, the hospital did not report the long-term results of radiation treatment, which undoubtedly were not so good. Surgery continued to show somewhat better results.

Palmer Hospital did not overlook patients needing terminal care. "There are in the Hospital today patients who have been in the institution for months and, in two instances, for years," reported Superintendent Hagen in 1928. As discussed before, the nursing care was extraordinary. One of Palmer's first patients was a minister, "unable to take a mouthful of food by himself, who for seven years had to be turned in bed every two hours," recorded an early history. "In all those years he was nursed with such care that he never had a bed sore or an accident of any kind."

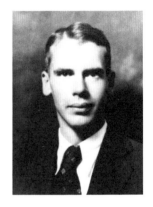

DR. SHIELDS WARREN, CA. 1918. *As the hospital's chief pathologist, Warren established the first unified department of pathology in Boston. A talented scientist, Warren became one of the hospital's most renowned staff members.*

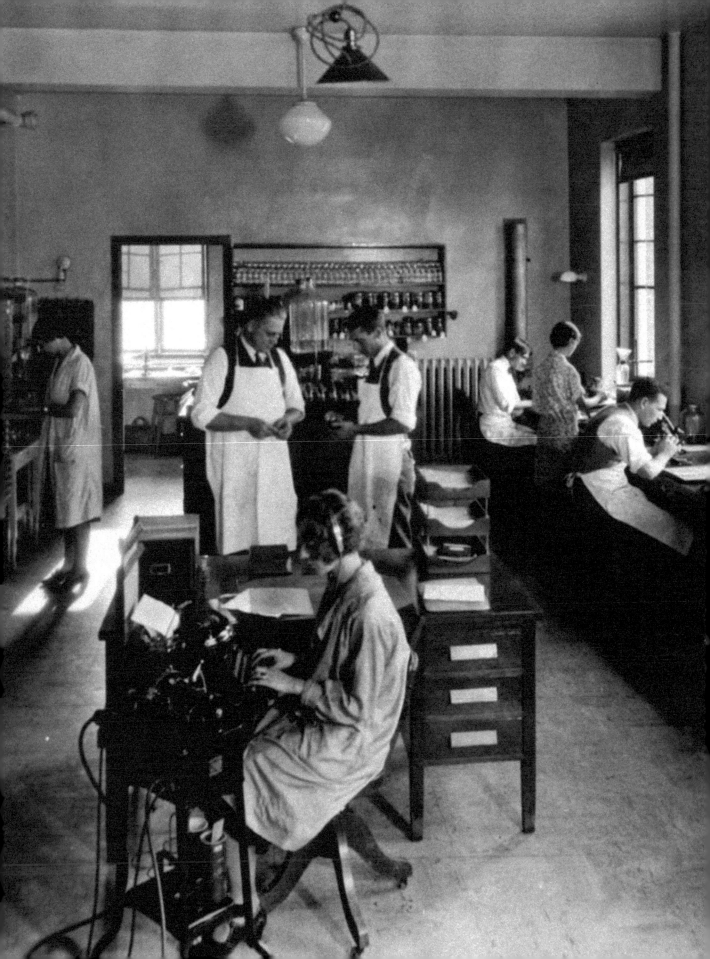

While the new Palmer Hospital reflected the Deaconess's growing emphasis on specialized care, it mirrored as well the institution's aspiration to be in the forefront of medicine and medical research, even though it was not an academic hospital per se. The religious and charitable impulses that had inspired the Deaconess's founding remained evident in the free care it provided to impecunious patients and in its Sunday prayer services. But in its club-like atmosphere, appointments, and private rooms, Palmer Hospital also had the aspect of an affluent private hospital. In fact, as epitomized by the new Palmer, the Deaconess had become an interesting hybrid, at once secular and religious, private and charitable, scientific and non-academic.

BY THE LATE 1920s, New England Deaconess Hospital had come to be dominated by several strong, successful, and visionary doctors. What had been true of the Deaconess in 1896 was unchanged in 1928, however — skilled doctors came and gladly remained because of the dedicated, compassionate, and competent care that its nurses gave to their patients. The early deaconesses themselves had established a high standard of patient care that continued to be rigorously taught in the professional school of nursing and on the floors. The deaconess legacy, reinforced by an ongoing deaconess presence, was already deeply woven into the hospital's fabric.

PALMER LABORATORY, CA. 1927. *Headed by pathologist Shields Warren, the Palmer Laboratory was located between two major operating rooms. Palmer staff members were able to complete frozen section diagnoses on tumors in four to five minutes.*

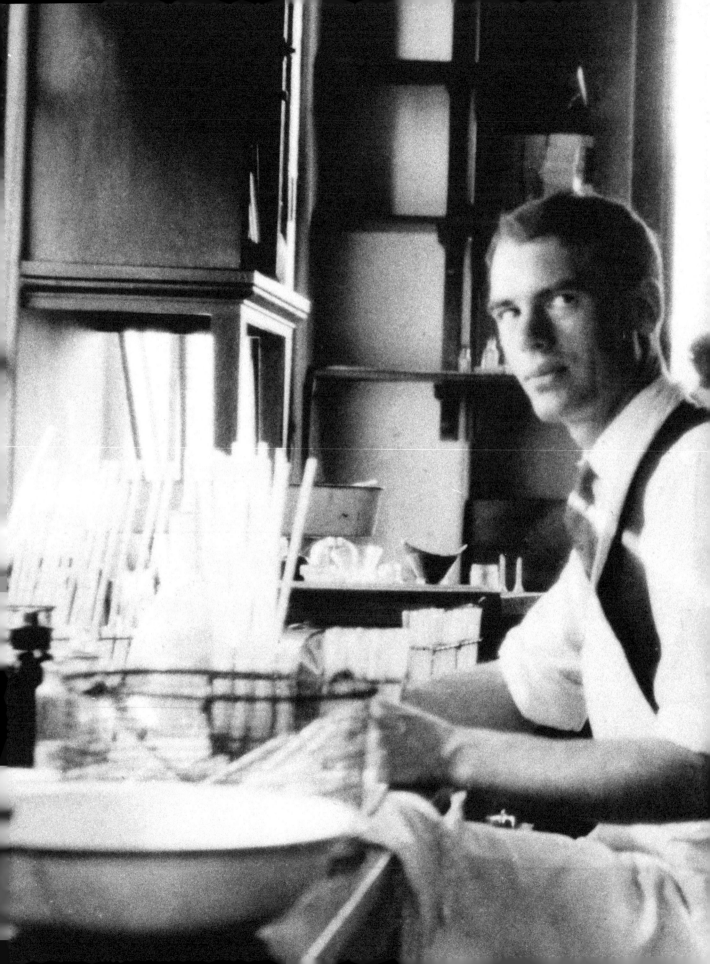

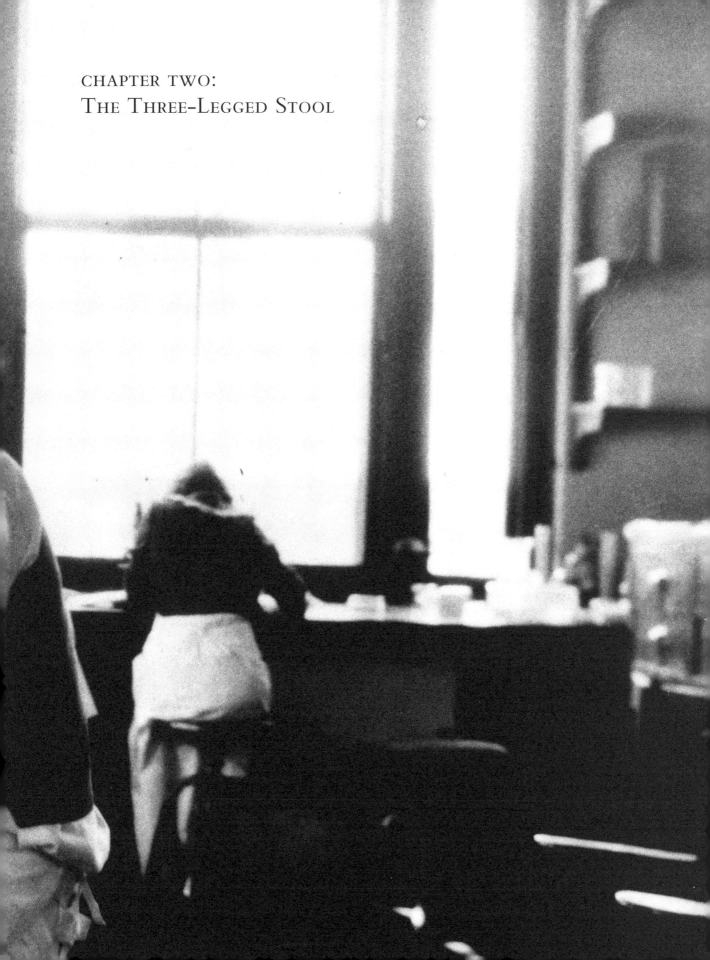

CHAPTER TWO:
The Three-Legged Stool

Overleaf:

Dr. Shields Warren in the Pathology Lab, ca. 1930. As the first permanent staff member of the reorganized Deaconess Hospital (which included Palmer Memorial), Warren headed the hospital's various laboratories, including pathology, chemical, metabolic, and electrocardio- graphic. In his long and varied career, Warren pursued many professional roles — as a busy practicing pathologist; active researcher in the fields of diabetes, thyroid disease, and cancer; pioneer investigator in atomic energy and medicine; and international authority on the effects of atomic radiation on humans. In addition, Warren trained more than 250 practicing pathologists. He was the recipient of many prestigious professional honors including the Enrico Fermi Award and the Einstein Medal and Award.

CHAPTER TWO:
THE THREE-LEGGED STOOL

In 1929, New England Deaconess Hospital broke away from the
Deaconess Association but not from the Methodist Church. Over
the next two decades, Deaconess Hospital developed a more modern,
elaborate, and centralized management, while balkanization of the
medical staff became an increasingly common theme. Despite constraints
imposed first by the Depression and then by World War II, the
Deaconess actually flourished and expanded during the 1930s and 1940s,
due largely to its renowned specialty clinics and successful independent
practitioners as well as its excellent nursing service and patient care.

SEPARATION AND A NEW SUPERINTENDENT

In the spring of 1929 New England Deaconess Hospital was separately
incorporated, as stated, "Its object shall be the treatment, care and relief
of sick and suffering persons and the maintenance of hospital and training
schools for nurses, and such other activities as may be related thereto."
A year later the Supreme Judicial Court of Massachusetts approved
the transfer of the hospital's land and buildings from the New England
Deaconess Association to the new corporation. In effect, the new
hospital corporation succeeded the New England Deaconess Association
as the hospital's owner and trustee.

Little documentary evidence is extant as to why this occurred,
and none of those with firsthand knowledge survives. Fortunately,
however, Robert D. (Don) Lowry, who joined the hospital as an administrator in 1946, and Richard (Dick) Lee, who went to work for the
New England Deaconess Association in 1951 and entered the hospital's
administrative staff in 1959, have recalled what their predecessors at
the hospital recounted. As reported, the Deaconess Association was using
surplus money from the hospital to support other Methodist institutions
in Massachusetts, including a children's camp in Attleboro, an old-age
home in Concord, and a nursing home in Natick. That practice precipitated a doctors' revolt led by Frank Lahey and Elliott Joslin, who wanted
any surplus generated by the hospital to be used there. Following a
dispute which left some hard feelings in its wake, the doctors prevailed
and the hospital was formally severed from the Association. The

separation did not mean that the hospital ceased to have a strong Methodist affiliation. In fact, the hospital's bylaws required that a majority of the corporation's members belong to the Methodist Episcopal Church. The officers and trustees, including the president, William Rich, were prominent Methodist laymen, generally business people, who associated regularly with their counterparts at other Methodist institutions, including the Deaconess Association, Morgan Memorial, and Boston University. Stanley O. MacMullen, a key member of the Board of Trustees and later its president, for example, was in the insurance business; his partner in the insurance industry, a fellow Methodist, served on the Deaconess Association's board. Not all trustees were Methodists, however. Francis W. (Frank) Capper, who was an Episcopalian and a banker at Boston Safe Deposit Company, became a trustee in 1932 and treasurer in 1934, serving very competently in that position for the next eighteen years.

At the time of the separation, the Board of Trustees also hired a new superintendent for the hospital, Warren F. Cook, an ordained Methodist minister with a doctorate in divinity, who was known as "Dr. Cook." He succeeded Caroline Jackson, a deaconess, who had followed Adeliza Betts as superintendent and served in that position for six years. The son of a minister, Cook was born in Eureka, Kansas, in 1883 and grew up in Kansas and Colorado. Coincidentally, Cook's father had been ordained by Shields Warren's grandfather, William Fairfield Warren, and named his son for him. Cook worked his way through college in part by playing professional baseball and by coaching his school team.

After completing college in Kansas, Cook studied at Yale Divinity School and Hartford Theological Seminary. During the First World War, he went to France with a group of speakers for the Y.M.C.A., and after the war, assumed a pulpit in Montclair, New Jersey. While there, he became involved in the Methodist Hospital in Brooklyn, New York. Fearing the death of the administrator, that hospital's board asked Cook to serve as assistant director and groomed him to advance when the time came. The administrator endured, however, and Cook remained assistant director for six years, when he was asked to become superintendent at New England Deaconess.

An upbeat, vigorous, and athletic man, Cook played golf and tennis and belonged to the hospital's bowling team. Although the focus of his career shifted, he had received no formal training in administration and retained his ministerial style. "The spirit which manifests itself in doctor, nurse and employee toward patient and visitor can and should reveal the life of the Great Physician," Cook wrote in the hospital's 1930 report. "Certainly, this spirit is nearest to the ideal when it manifests itself toward the poor."

Cook was a fluent speaker and writer who believed that the hospital benefited from favorable publicity and good public relations. He himself developed a colorful speech on "The Mystery and Romance of Radium," which brought attention to the hospital's having the largest supply of radium — two grams — in New England and one of the most advanced emanation plants in the world for deriving radon gas from radium. He gave versions of this speech to civic, fraternal, religious, and women's organizations throughout New England; it was also broadcast over the radio. Though radium and radon gas were at the time popular methods for the treatment of cancer, leading scientific experts recognized their limited effectiveness. Nevertheless, at the time, these therapies had considerable appeal to cancer victims, who saw them as desirable alternatives to surgery.

Cook initiated an in-house department of public relations and hired external public relations experts in conjunction with fund-raising drives. The hospital's gift shop expanded business and began to sell picture postcards of the Deaconess, which have since become collector's items. Cook became active in professional organizations, including the association of Boston hospital superintendents, and the New England and Massachusetts hospital associations, both of which he served as president. He also joined the American College of Hospital Administrators, which was formed in 1933 independent of the American Hospital Association. Cook's participation in these groups provided him with useful information about how other hospitals were run and gave him opportunities to spread the good word about the Deaconess.

When Cook became superintendent, Deaconess Hospital comprised 225 beds and its buildings had a book value of $1.8 million. In a talk he gave to department heads six years later, Cook compared the hospital to a large hotel, except that the guests did not leave their beds. During this period the laundry processed 30,000 to 40,000 pieces a week, the chemical laboratory completed more than 100,000 tests a year, and the pharmacy bustled. Cook's own time was consumed by meetings — with department heads, trustees, Executive Committee members, prospective donors, lawyers, individual employees, and patients. He was always available to hear doctors' complaints

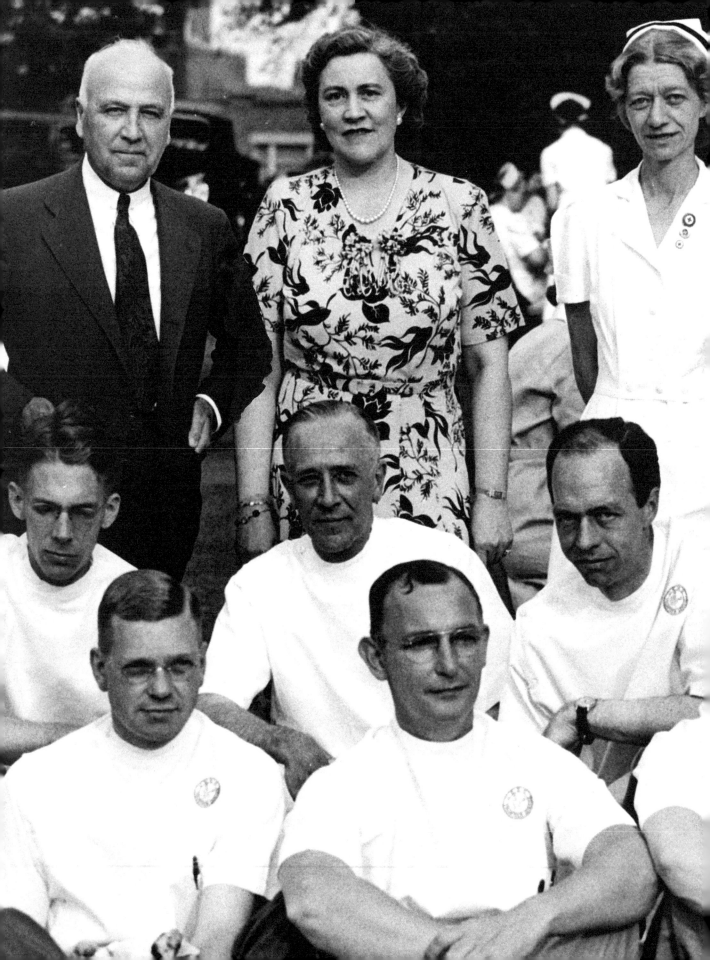

and suggestions. In addition, he represented the hospital externally, kept up a busy speaking schedule, and regularly participated in prayer services at the Deaconess nursing school.

Cook's activism and businesslike approach apparently did not meet with total acceptance by the medical staff. Acting as chairman of the hospital's combined staffs, Shields Warren reported to the Executive Committee a resolution that had been unanimously passed on January 28, 1935: "The Staff of the New England Deaconess Hospital . . . believe that one of the features of this hospital which has made it successful and agreeable is the family-like relationship between the Trustees, the Hospital Administration, and the Staff. The Staff feel that views held and the recommendations made by Dr. Cook are diametrically opposed to the views of the Staff. Because of Dr. Cook's known attitude toward institutionalizing this hospital, the Staff suggests careful consideration by the Trustees of Dr. Cook's value to the hospital."

The mistrust was not confined to the Deaconess. Doctors nationally were feeling threatened by the new breed of ambitious, non-medical hospital administrators who were beginning to emerge in these years. To doctors, hospital administrators could appear as self-perpetuating empire-builders and a threat to the physicians' power. In his presidential address to the New England Surgical Association in 1932, for example, Frank Lahey cautioned against the growing authority of hospital superintendents. He pointed out that he himself had not experienced this phenomenon in his own hospitals, but this was three years before the Deaconess staff tried to get Cook removed. "The proper hospital situation is, in my opinion," said Lahey, "a relationship in which the doctors on a hospital staff are closest to the trustees and the hospital superintendents are under the direction of the hospital staff or on the same executive level as the staff, rather than one in which the staff is under the direction of the superintendent."

Even though Cook was a minister and had not received formal training in accounting, business, or industrial engineering, as had some of his fellow administrators, he did share many of the new breed's values and priorities. Cook established, for example, a Department of Social Service in 1933 under Gertrude Jameson. While this decision was in keeping with modern medical administration, doctors sometimes viewed

WARREN F. COOK, CA. 1945. Cook assumed the Deaconess directorship in 1929 and remained until 1954, overseeing the hospital's growth from 225 to 375 beds. A professional baseball player with the Kansas City Blues early in his career and an ordained minister, Cook came to the Deaconess from the New York Methodist Hospital in Brooklyn. Cook (back row, left) posed for this photograph with Constance Learned, Director of Volunteer Services (center), staff nurse Muriel Lund (right), and members of the Medical Aides, seventeen men specially trained in patient care who served the hospital during World War II.

the department as either an encroachment or an unnecessary encumbrance.
The next year Cook hired a financial assistant, William B. Nash, to help him
and the volunteer treasurer, Frank Capper. Gradually, under Cook's direction,
the non-medical administration began to grow.

Only a week before the doctors adopted their unanimous resolution,
Cook had made three suggestions to the board's Executive Committee that
apparently raised the doctors' ire. First, he proposed setting aside certain wards
at the Deaconess for poorer patients, just as was done at Palmer Hospital,
"where the administration with the doctor shall decide and collect both the
hospital bill and the doctor's fee." Cook noted that this was common practice
in most hospitals, including the Baker Memorial at Massachusetts General
Hospital. "I think we should also prepare our minds for some prepayment
[insurance] plan for hospital bills whereby poorer patients can take care of their
unexpected hospital bills," Cook stated. Such plans had not yet won acceptance in New England and were anathema to the American Medical Association. Morris Fishbein, the crusading editor of the *Journal of the American Medical
Association,* had helped unify medical opinion against group prepayment,
characterizing it as a step toward socialism and communism. But by the end
of 1934, following the establishment of the Associated Hospital Service Plan
of New York [City], hospital insurance was becoming a national movement.
Cook acknowledged that the Deaconess could not act by itself, "but the
time is fast approaching when hospitals will have to do something of this kind
for the poor patients or they will be forced to do it by the government."

Cook's third recommendation may have provoked the medical
staff most of all. Possibly through his involvement in professional associations,
Cook had learned that the Deaconess was not "organized as the average
Class A hospital," which did not elect staff doctors as members of their boards
of trustees. Most Class A hospitals, he pointed out, had a board separate and
distinct from their hospital staff. A conference committee, composed of
members from each group, worked out "inter-related problems." "Under the
present arrangement," Cook asserted, "you have members on your Board
of Trustees who are both advocate and judge."

In response to Shields Warren's letter, the Executive Committee,
which itself included one doctor, Leland McKittrick, the chief surgeon at
Palmer Hospital, unanimously agreed with the doctors' encomium about the

value of a "family-like relationship" and continued, "earnestly hopes that this pleasant and cordial relationship between the members of the Staff and the members of the Hospital Administration and the Trustees shall continue to grow and increase." Soon thereafter the Executive Committee met with Warren, Lahey, and Joslin as well as with Cook, and appointed a three-person committee to try to resolve the situation.

Several weeks later, on the recommendation of the special committee, the Executive Committee voted to retain Cook, with Miss Mabel Eager and Mrs. Roscoe Carter, two Methodist benefactors, dissenting. According to Don Lowry, Cook's being a Methodist minister gave him a great deal of credibility with Stanley MacMullen and other trustees and was probably what saved his job. However, the Executive Committee did instruct Cook to arrange for weekly meetings with department heads and to define the duties of Sadie Hagen, a deaconess who had been Palmer's superintendent and then assistant superintendent of the Deaconess following Cook's arrival. Hagen and Cook evidently had not hit it off, which had probably added to his troubles. Indeed, when Hagen retired in 1943 after forty-two years of service at the Deaconess, Cook complimented her in a left-handed way that also hinted at his own earlier failure to appreciate fully her popularity and influence: "While Miss Hagen is not a trained nurse or a formally trained administrator, she is a grand person, with personality and judgment and a great liking for people which has made her of inestimable help in the Hospital."

That Cook survived the attempted purge in 1935 suggests that doctors did not, in fact, have complete and total control of the Deaconess. Although the hospital continued to have a number of doctors on its Board of Trustees and even one on its Executive Committee, the lay trustees had evidently begun to assert their responsibility for the welfare of the institution as a whole, most particularly for its finances and non-medical administration. Lay trustees and the administrators who were answerable to them, of course, desired friendly, cooperative relationships with doctors and fully appreciated their importance. But they also began to recognize that doctors could be self-interested and unconcerned about the hospital's finances and its overall mission.

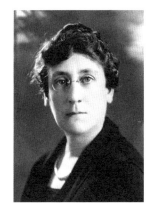

SADIE A. HAGEN, CA. 1930. *A native of Ireland, Hagen attended the Deaconess Training School before beginning a forty-two-year association with the Deaconess. After serving as superintendent of the New England [Deaconess] Home and Palmer Memorial Hospital, Hagen was appointed assistant superintendent of New England Deaconess Hospital in 1929 and remained in that position until her retirement in 1943.*

FLOURISHING THROUGH THE DEPRESSION

The Depression evidently underscored to the trustees their need to keep a close eye on the hospital's bottom line. As the economy declined in 1930 and 1931, the Deaconess's census fell too and so did revenues, contributions, and bequests; simultaneously, the number of non-paying and part-pay patients rose, a 15 percent increase in 1931 alone. More than most religious or voluntary hospitals, the Deaconess had financed its expansion in the 1920s through debt. More commonly, religious and voluntary hospitals expanded only after they had sufficient capital in hand.

In contrast to some of its Boston counterparts, moreover, the Deaconess had only a modest endowment. Its board was composed of self-made Methodist businessmen, not people with inherited wealth. As entrepreneurs themselves, they had not been afraid to let the hospital finance its expansion through debt. As long as the economy was expanding, interest charges were not a major concern. But after the economy began to contract, debt service became burdensome.

Chastened, the trustees adopted a policy in 1930 "not to erect buildings without funds to do the same." In 1931 the hospital had an operating deficit (whose size was not divulged) which Cook pointed out in the annual report was only slightly larger than the interest charges it was paying on its mortgages. "This indebtedness is a millstone about our necks," he wrote, "and must be moved before we can make progress. Because of these interest charges we have not been able to pay our bills promptly, and therefore have been unable to take advantage of trade discounts."

In early 1931, evidently short of operating funds, the hospital secured a half-million-dollar mortgage from National Shawmut Bank of Boston at the rate of 6 percent, payable semi-annually. The hospital also had substantial loans from the First National Bank of Boston. According to a story that Dick Lee later heard, sometime in the 1930s both banks forgave a portion of the loans. Unfortunately, verification of such acts of bank philanthropy has not shown up in hospital records, though there is an indication that both banks did reschedule payments in 1935.

What is certain is that in 1931 and 1932 the hospital tried to cut costs wherever it could. Wage reductions of 5 to 10 percent were instituted, free work was provided only to the extent that the hospital had received endowment or contributions for that purpose, and cafeteria service replaced waitress-served meals for nurses. In addition, the hospital enhanced revenues by improving its pharmacy, which sold to the public. In fact, only a quarter of the pharmacy's sales were to inpatients. The second floor of Palmer Hospital, previously burdened with empty beds, was converted into a low-priced section accommodating twenty-eight patients. Outpatient fees were lowered from $5.00 to $1.50, the same rate charged by state clinics. A large, anonymous gift underwrote charitable cases in Palmer, with doctors donating their services. Treasurer Frank Capper is reported to have played a major role in engineering the hospital's financial recovery. In 1934, the hospital's census and income returned to their pre-Depression levels. Patient income increased 20 percent between 1933 and 1934 alone. Indebtedness was reduced by $52,000, endowments increased by $65,000, all current bills were paid, including $48,000 in interest, while $44,000 was spent on improvements. In that year, the hospital provided $63,650 in free care.

Among hospitals nationwide, the major casualties of the Depression were small single-specialty and small proprietary-general hospitals. Large, nonprofit, voluntary hospitals, including religious institutions, which had been the largest providers of hospital care in the 1920s, retained their dominant positions in the 1930s. For New England Deaconess, as for other strong voluntary institutions, the Depression only marked a temporary and fairly short-lived setback.

DESPITE THE DEPRESSION, the number of hospital beds in the United States actually increased during the 1930s. To some extent, expansion was fueled by advances in medicine and surgery, in medical technology and pharmacology, and by the continued growth of specialization. But it was also supported by government, specifically by President Franklin D. Roosevelt's New Deal. The Works Progress Administration (WPA) spent more than $77 million on hospital construction in the United States between 1935 and 1938. In Boston, for example, the Public Works Administration (PWA) funded a modern, ten-story building at Boston City Hospital. Both the PWA and the WPA focused on municipal, psychiatric, and tuberculosis hospitals. Voluntary hospitals rarely benefited; indeed, they began to fear government encroachment. Hence, such

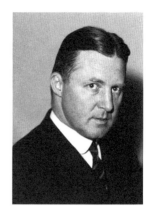

FRANCIS W. CAPPER, CA. 1934. *Capper first came to the Deaconess as a patient in the 1920s then rose to corporation member in the 1930s, hospital treasurer in 1934, president of the corporation in 1956, and chairman of the board in 1964. He is credited with helping to ensure the hospital's financial health during the Depression. A surgery lectureship in Capper's honor was established in 1978, a lasting tribute to his long service to the hospital.*

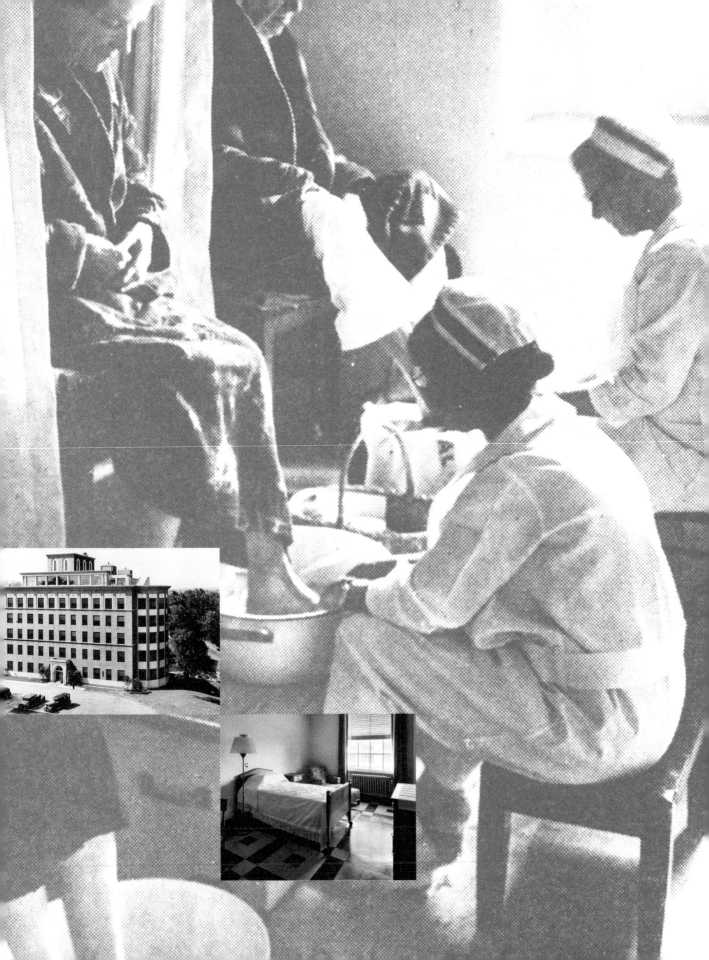

hospitals started to emphasize that they also provided a social service through their care of indigent patients. As institutions serving the community, they too could stake a claim to government support.

Hospitals that had building plans on the drawing boards at the outset of the Depression had to decide whether to proceed. Of course, in 1929 and 1930 no one knew how long the economic downturn would last and many, from President Herbert Hoover on down, hoped for the best. Meanwhile, construction costs were dropping significantly, which offered an inducement to expand. Indeed, this was exactly the Deaconess's situation in 1928 vis-à-vis a building for diabetes and other chronic diseases made possible by a $250,000 bequest from George F. Baker, a prominent New York banker. In 1930 the architectural firm of Coolidge Shepley Bulfinch and Abbott was engaged to draw up plans. Two years later, George B. H. Macomber and Company bid $297,562 to construct the new building, $86,000 *less* than had originally been anticipated.

Even so, the trustees were understandably wary since the hospital was heavily in debt and was experiencing operating deficits. Reportedly, there was a test of wills between Joslin and reluctant trustees, with Joslin prevailing since he actually controlled the securities that Baker had donated. Unfortunately, Joslin sold these securities at rock-bottom prices to pay for construction. In authorizing building to proceed, the Board of Trustees stipulated that the money be in hand and accepted Joslin's guarantee of $15,000 a year for twenty years to cover overhead. The written agreement indicated that Joslin had shown the finance committee pledges and extracts from wills worth approximately $518,000. Though the committee acknowledged that the pledges were not guarantees, it was willing to accept them as ample protection for the hospital.

The George F. Baker Clinic, a six-story building that arose on land Joslin had bought on Pilgrim Road in 1932, was dedicated in March 1934, but was not fully in service for another two years. As director of the first center in the United States devoted to the care, study, and treatment of diabetic patients, Joslin hoped that the new clinic would be a model for others to come. Baker included a dental room, chemical laboratory, administrative offices, classrooms for teaching diabetic patients, and private and semi-private patient rooms.

VIEWS OF THE GEORGE F. BAKER CLINIC, CA. 1935. Designed by architects Coolidge Shepley Bulfinch and Abbott of Boston, the Baker Clinic housed both the research and treatment facilities for the work of Joslin and his associates. The clinic's six floors (five stories plus basement) included more than a dozen laboratories, a foot room for treating conditions common to diabetics, a large class or demonstration area, rooms for forty-seven patients, and a penthouse gymnasium for children. The original Baker bequest designated that the money was to be used for "chronic disease should the need for diabetic treatment pass."

The new Baker facilities also included a foot room devoted to treatment of foot problems such as infection and gangrene, common side effects of diabetes. In 1928 Joslin had engineered the appointment of John F. Kelly, a podiatrist, as consultant to the foot-care clinic at the Deaconess. Kelly, a graduate of the School of Podiatry at the University of Massachusetts, was reportedly the first podiatrist appointed to the staff of a major hospital in the United States. He was subsequently joined by I. Malcolm Humphrey, a graduate of the Beacon Institute of Podiatry and Temple University's School of Podiatry. In effect, Joslin, Kelly, and Humphrey laid the foundation for hospital-based podiatry in this country.

Joslin's assistants at Baker included Howard Root, Priscilla White, Alexander Marble, C. Cabell Bailey, and Allen Joslin, Elliott's son. Thanks in part to their collaborative efforts, the care of diabetic coma improved significantly in the 1930s. Baker Clinic also included a research laboratory where Marble carried out important metabolic and other research, some involving experiments with diabetes in animals. As officials routinely pointed out, however, practically all research conducted at the Deaconess was supported by outside funds, not by the hospital.

To be sure, not every important development in diabetic research or treatment occurred at Deaconess Hospital, nor every advance associated with Joslin. Priscilla White, a 1923 graduate of Tufts Medical School, was appointed to the Deaconess staff in 1924 when she joined Joslin's practice. An important pioneer in juvenile diabetes, White vastly improved the safety of pregnancy for diabetic women and their fetuses. The Deaconess, however, lacked an obstetrical department, and although it admitted some children, there were other Boston hospitals that specialized in pediatrics. As a result, many of White's hospitalized patients went elsewhere.

In time, the Baker Clinic building came to be regarded by administrators as a serious error in design — its floors were too small and therefore much too costly to staff. No one was ever able to determine the separate costs of running the building, however, so Joslin's so-called "guarantee fund" was never called upon to pay for any shortfall, though Joslin did account for additional gifts to the hospital. Partly because of the large number of private rooms, Baker was thought of as a "ritzy" part of the hospital. Baker even had a doorman, who wore a suit and a cap with the initials NEDH on its front. One day, the story goes, a little boy whose mother was a patient asked the doorman what the letters stood for and he answered, "Nobody ever dies here."

BY 1934, WHEN THE BAKER CLINIC OPENED, the Deaconess was recovering from the financial impact of the early Depression. The following year Cook reported the largest census in the hospital's history. "Many times we have taxed the capacity of the hospital and turned patients away," he observed. "During the first eleven months we equalled the census of twelve months last." Utilization would never slacken through the rest of the decade. In 1939, for example, Cook reported an effective occupancy rate of approximately 94 percent; the Deaconess had to refuse 1,591 patients. That same year fifteen hospitals in the Boston metropolitan area showed an average occupancy rate of 81 percent, which was considered an efficient operating level. Ninety percent and above was a real strain, but it was to become the norm at the Deaconess for many years to come.

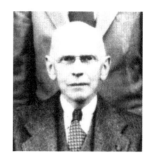

MEMBERS OF DR. JOSLIN'S TEAM, CA. 1950. *From top: Dr. Elliott P. Joslin, Dr. Allen Joslin, Dr. Robert F. Bradley, Jr., Dr. Priscilla White, Dr. Alexander Marble, and Dr. Howard F. Root.*

As in the 1920s, the Deaconess's beds were utilized by patients who had been admitted by doctors who were independent practitioners, or those either affiliated with the Lahey Clinic or members of Joslin's private practice. In terms of its patient base, the Deaconess was therefore a kind of "three-legged stool." Because two of those legs were quite specialized — the Joslin's in diabetes and the Lahey Clinic's in a growing number of areas — the Deaconess itself became known as a specialty, not general, hospital.

Since so many of its patients had originally been referred to one of the hospital's affiliated specialists by their local physicians, it was vital that their experience at the Deaconess be satisfactory. If a patient went home and complained to his or her doctor about surly or indifferent nurses, about bad food or unpleasant surroundings, the physician would be much less inclined to refer patients in the future. (That would also be the outcome if the specialist "stole" the patient from the referring physician, something which Lahey and Joslin doctors were careful to avoid.) Its staff physicians, likewise, expected the hospital to be well run and to treat patients kindly.

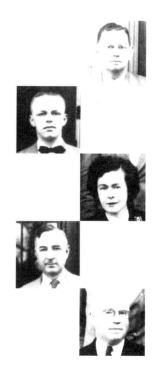

Although no surveys were taken, the fact that the Deaconess operated at capacity suggests that patient satisfaction was high. The average length of stay in the late 1930s and early 1940s was approximately thirteen days, which was consistent with the average over the previous twenty years. Doctors who worked at the hospital in the 1930s and 1940s and who have been interviewed for this book uniformly praised the hospital's administration, nursing, and patient care.

After World War II, Warren Cook published a booklet of unsolicited letters he had received from patients and their families, which he titled *Proof*. The writers spanned the social and economic scale. "We were with you eight long weeks and I shall never forget how kind everyone was to us," wrote the wife of a patient from Hartford. Her husband had been too ill to know or care where he was, but she had been full of indescribable lonesomeness when they arrived. "From the time the first nurse spoke [to me] until we both left the hospital, never was such kindness, courtesy, and thoughtfulness shown to any millionaire patient."

A Methodist minister from the Tremont Street Methodist Church in Boston expressed his appreciation for the splendid free care received by an impecunious church member, who had been hospitalized twice with cancer: "The kindly care she received could not have been better if she had paid the highest price in a private room." Louis Fabian Bachrach, the famous portrait photographer, observed appreciatively that his wife had "been in a number of hospitals in her life and has never received the treatment that she did there." A Florida man wrote, "I believe with all my heart that your hospital is the best in the country." And Boston physician Louis S. Chase paid tribute, "From the point of vantage of one who has worked closely in dozens of hospitals and has had the opportunity to see the working of hospitals on several occasions in the role of patient, my brief sojourn at the New England Deaconess Hospital was especially gratifying. All departments seemed to be competing for highest honors of efficiency — from the kitchen with its excellent menus (plus choice!), maids, student nurses to supervising nurses, and physicians to consulting staff."

PROFESSIONAL NURSING TRAINING AND PRACTICE

By the end of the Depression, as the nursing staff became fully secularized and professionalized, few deaconesses remained. The last nurse-deaconess may have been Nannie C. Peterson, who was well known for her strong opinions. "It was reported to the [nurse training school] committee that Miss Nannie Peterson, a graduate nurse, had upon several occasions been known to make adverse and destructive criticism of the hospital and the training school management," the minutes of that committee noted in 1932. "The secretary was instructed to write Miss Peterson in reference to this matter."

Internist Robert (Bob) Brownlee, who first came to the Deaconess as a student house officer in 1936, vividly recalled Peterson's telling him that she had been the night superintendent of a tent hospital during the great flu epidemic. "Dr. Brownlee," she said, "people died all over the world, but nobody died in my hospital." "Nannie," Brownlee thought to himself, "they just didn't dare!" Later he cared for Peterson's brother-in-law, who came to the hospital suffering from an intestinal obstruction. According to Brownlee, Peterson became upset because she thought his abdominal distension would have been relieved by an old-fashioned flaxseed poultice. None of the nurses even knew what a flaxseed poultice was by that time.

Traditionally, nursing was seen as a worthy profession that also enabled women to earn a living, albeit a very modest one. It has been said that nursing appealed to women's ideals and to their sense of service. During the Depression, hospital diploma programs decreased nationally, from more than 2,286 in 1929 to 1,472 in 1936. At the same time, the number of collegiate programs, which usually entailed two years of general education either before or after a three-year hospital diploma program, began to grow — increasing to 7 by 1936.

Even before the Depression, the nursing profession was experiencing difficulties as a result of an overexpansion of training schools, too many of which were substandard, and an oversupply of nurses. The Depression exacerbated the situation as the number of hospitals contracted and private-duty nursing opportunities shrank. A Boston nursing registry in 1931 reported members asking for work; the following year they sought financial assistance. According to one source, 60 percent of all nurses in the United States were unemployed by 1933.

At the Deaconess, as at many hospitals, nurses' salaries were reduced in the depths of the Depression and were not fully restored until the end of the 1930s. As a way of increasing the number of nurses who could be employed, the Deaconess, like many hospitals, indeed like many different kinds of employers in the Depression, instituted the eight-hour workday. Despite having their salaries reduced, however,

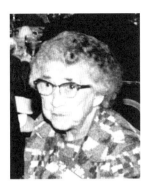

THE HOSPITAL'S LAST SURVIVING DEACONESS, NANNIE C. PETERSON. *In her forty-seven years at Deaconess Hospital, Peterson served as staff nurse, private duty nurse, and head of the operating room nursing staff. Born in Sweden, Peterson graduated from the Deaconess Training School and performed mission work before completing her studies as a member of the Deaconess Nursing School Class of 1915. She died at the Deaconess in 1980 at the age of ninety-eight.*

all staff nurses at the Deaconess generously contributed five days' pay in 1933 to the Boston Emergency Relief Fund.

IN THE EARLY 1930s, the Deaconess nursing school admitted about fifty students a year, half in September and half in January. At least that number was needed every year to cover the hospital's staffing needs. Until 1938 students were on duty eight hours every day of the year, except for a short vacation in the summer; in 1938, the school began to give students the equivalent of one day off per week. In addition, nursing students had four hours of class a week, some of which took place at Simmons College or was given by Simmons instructors; they also had to find time to study. During the second half of the 1930s, the total number of students declined from 150 to 105. The graduate or staff nurses at the hospital expanded commensurately, from 16 in 1935 to 90 in 1939, a dramatic increase, but in line with national trends. Over the same time period, the number of head nurses increased from 16 to 22; orderlies and attendants, who came under the direction of the nursing department, decreased from 22 to 16.

As before, the school had high standards, meeting or exceeding those set by nursing and accrediting organizations, and it demanded much of its students. "During the year, 12 students have withdrawn from the school, four for personal reasons, and the others because they lacked the peculiar [sic] characteristics which must be present in certain proportions in order to successfully meet the demands made upon the nurse of today," Marjorie B. Davis, the superintendent of nurses, observed in 1938.

Indeed, the Deaconess Hospital School of Nursing required total commitment and dedication. Students were not allowed to be married. Relatively few of the staff or graduate nurses were wed and practically none of the supervisors was. Nursing director Lois M. Preston, who matriculated at the school in January 1938, later recalled asking Miss Davis permission to attend Rainbow, a Masonic girls organization, on one Thursday night a month. "Do you want to be a nurse or do you want to stay in Rainbow?" Davis asked. Preston had to give up her night out. Another alumna from this period did not return until her twenty-fifth reunion, it was later recalled, because she had not gotten over a painful experience she had as a student. Her brother had died and the school's director forced her to make the horrible choice of attending his funeral or remaining in school.

Bob Brownlee recalled sometimes encountering a student nurse sobbing in the nurses' station because a very demanding night supervisor had ordered her to redo a chart. "She [the supervisor] required these student nurses to make perfect dots of each temperature, blood pressure, and pulse reading and to draw a line with a ruler from the center of that dot to the center of the next dot four hours later and any smudge or failure to make the dot round would mean redoing the whole chart at two or three o'clock in the morning." Such attention to detail was taken for granted as part of the discipline of Deaconess nurses, just as starched uniforms and proper caps. (Nursing was hierarchical and this was reflected in their attire.) Although the field had become more technically sophisticated and professionalized over the previous thirty years, it remained clearly subordinate to the medical profession. Indeed, it was customary at the time for a nurse to rise when a doctor entered a room.

The school's ethos emphasized superior, not merely adequate, nursing. Consequently, its graduates usually were at an advantage in the tight job market of the 1930s, even at a great distance from Boston. Don Lowry's first awareness of Deaconess Hospital came in the late 1930s when he heard a nursing superintendent in a California hospital tell her assistant that she was not interested in interviewing any new nurses because she was fully staffed. She would, however, make an exception were a Deaconess graduate to come along. It seemed that she had in the past hired three Deaconess nurses and they had all proven to be superior; she was even ready to lay off one of her current staff if a Deaconess graduate appeared.

Not all Deaconess nurses were graduates of its nursing school. Marjorie Davis, for example, the school's superintendent and the hospital's director of nursing from 1936 to 1944, had trained at Johns Hopkins. Margaret Shrader, her successor, had also been trained elsewhere — at Columbia Presbyterian and Boston University. The hospital employed two male nurses for urological patients, and they were certainly not Deaconess graduates since the school did not admit men. But the hospital did hire many of its own graduates and they rose up the ranks to staff nurse, assistant head nurse, head nurse, supervisor, assistant director, and even director. Some alumnae of course went to other hospitals, often because they wanted to have a new experience or live elsewhere. But it was also quite common for them to return to the Deaconess at some point in their careers.

Many Deaconess nursing students came from small New England cities and towns, and the school continued to have a Protestant dimension; attendance at chapel service was required. The school's credo in the 1930s called for "ministering to the sick of all races and creeds without preference." Although people of all kinds were welcomed as patients, the school's staff, students, and alumnae opposed admitting Catholics and Jews to the school itself. An exception was apparently made for a German-Jewish refugee during the Second World War. The school, however, rejected a clergyman's request to admit two Japanese-American students in 1943 "on the basis that we are dealing with sick people, our students affiliate at other hospitals and we must not place ourselves in the position of creating discord or embarrassment." It was, unfortunately, one among many instances in wartime America when civil rights fell victim to anti-Japanese hysteria.

When a Catholic nurse's aide who had worked at the hospital during the war applied for admission in 1945, it prompted a debate within the school's advisory committee about its Protestants-only policy. Warren Cook favored dropping the restriction, but the school's faculty voted twenty-seven to three to retain it. By 1951, however, the practice was modified. Public attitudes about such restrictions were changing, as reflected in the establishment of the Massachusetts Commission Against Discrimination in the late 1940s. The school's 1951 catalogue read: "No discrimination is made, regardless of race, color, or creed. However, the emphasis of the School is primarily Protestant; it is expected that all students will conform to its program." Thus, non-Protestants were admitted, but were still expected to attend chapel services. Similarly, although no documentary evidence has surfaced to prove the point, individual physicians have recalled the existence of barriers to the hospital's staff well into the 1940s, though no such practices had been evident in the hospital's earliest days. Reportedly, a powerful member of the independent medical staff blocked staff appointments because of ethnic or religious orientation. Such discrimination was hardly unique to the Deaconess; staffs at other leading hospitals also engaged in this kind of prejudicial behavior.

BEFORE THE INTRODUCTION OF NEW DRUGS in the late 1930s, nursing care often made the difference between life and death. Nurses were responsible, among other things, for positioning patients correctly, for closely monitoring and controlling their temperatures and conditions, and for carefully dressing and draining wounds. A diabetic patient might stay in the hospital for a year while an ulcer or wound healed. "The bedside care was superb," reflected Brownlee, "in a way compensating for what we couldn't do in those days, although we thought we were doing wonderful things."

In time powerful new families of drugs began to enter the arsenal of medicine — sulfanilamide in 1937, followed by other sulfa drugs in ensuing years. Penicillin, restricted for military use at first, was tightly rationed to civilian hospitals before becoming more readily available in 1945 and 1946. Other antibiotics followed. But the introduction of sulfa and the other new wonder drugs hardly rendered nurses superfluous. On the contrary, these medications required extremely careful patient-monitoring because of their side-effects and possible toxicity. Good nursing remained critical to the care of the hospital's many diabetic patients; nurses who concentrated on diabetic care became knowledgeable about diet and other aspects of controlling the disease and then were responsible for imparting this information to patients. Moreover, as surgeons at the Deaconess performed increasingly difficult procedures, operating-room nurses provided essential support. Recovery rooms had not yet been devised and patients went directly from the operating room back to their beds. Unlike Boston's teaching hospitals, the Deaconess had no residents, and it was largely up to the floor nurses, including students, to attend to patients as they came out of anesthesia.

CULTIVATING MEDICAL TALENT

The Deaconess continued to have renowned doctors on its staff who, like the nurses, were devoted to patient care. Elliott Joslin and Frank Lahey, great figures and personalities each, were further developing their respective specialties in the 1930s and 1940s, which brought new medical and surgical talent to the Deaconess. The hospital also maintained high-caliber independent staff, and its pathology department excelled under Shields Warren.

In addition to providing clinical services, Joslin, Lahey, and Warren conducted research and directed fellowship programs although there was only an arms-length relationship between the hospital and Harvard, Tufts, or Boston University. Fellows and trainees had quite circumscribed patient responsibilities. In addition, a small number of Harvard medical students lived in surplus rooms in Palmer; six fourth-year students were paid a nominal sum to be "house officers." They assisted with certain night emergencies, took histories on new admissions, gave intravenous solutions, drew blood samples, and performed certain tests — nurses were at that time prohibited from doing many of these tasks.

One of Joslin's fellows was Deaconess internist L. Tillman McDaniel. In his fourth year at Harvard Medical School, McDaniel, a Texan and graduate of the University of Texas, enrolled in a well-known course in the instruction of diabetics, which Joslin had initiated. McDaniel had worked in Shields Warren's laboratory in his second year of medical school in 1933 and lived in a spare room in Palmer during his third and fourth years. Following a two-year internship at the University of Michigan, McDaniel was invited back by Howard Root for a two-year fellowship. After that he went to work as an assistant to Leroy Parkins, an internist on the Deaconess staff. In 1946, following wartime service, McDaniel established his own practice in Boston and applied for and received staff privileges at the Deaconess. His experience was not unusual; many Deaconess physicians and surgeons in the postwar period had some prior association with the hospital, either during medical school or later through a fellowship. The priority of both the specialty clinics and the independent staff, however, was patient care, not training either medical students or specialists.

IN 1932 LELAND MCKITTRICK succeeded his mentor, Daniel Fiske Jones, as surgeon-in-chief at Palmer Hospital. The son of a rural Wisconsin physician, McKittrick had graduated from the University of Wisconsin and Harvard Medical School. A gentleman, who could also be quite blunt, McKittrick recognized that he needed diversions to maintain his sense of humor and his dedication to patients. He carefully preserved time to go horseback riding, hunting and rowing, and to play squash. When a patient needed to be seen in the hospital, however, he was there.

Like Jones and Richardson before him, McKittrick was a renowned surgeon and teacher at Massachusetts General Hospital, with which he was closely identified. Although McKittrick placed quite a few of his private patients in the Deaconess, he also saw those who could not afford to pay either him or the hospital. (In the depths of the Depression, some of Palmer's private beds were converted to wards for cancer patients of limited means. In addition, Joslin and Root referred many diabetic patients to McKittrick, some of whom were indigent.)

A gifted and creative surgeon, McKittrick was a leader in the development of colon surgery and devised a new kind of ulcer surgery, the two-stage gastrectomy, which saved many lives in its day. His greatest fame, however, probably derived from his surgery on diabetics, and most of this work was concentrated at the Deaconess. Although his writings on colon and stomach procedures were usually coauthored with colleagues from Massachusetts General, McKittrick's papers on diabetic surgery were ordinarily written with Joslin physicians, which helped focus a spotlight on the Deaconess. In 1928, with Howard Root, he wrote a classic text, *Diabetic Surgery.* McKittrick also developed transmetatarsal amputation, which saved the legs of thousands of patients. Previously, most diabetics with serious ulcers or infections had required above-the-knee amputations.

McKittrick's contribution to diabetic surgery was all the more notable because he was a general, and not an orthopedic, surgeon. Before McKittrick became active in this area, diabetics had poor surgical experiences. Indeed, he began to achieve success where there had only been failure. In the 1930s McKittrick wrote that if some way of combating postoperative infections could be found, diabetics would have much higher survival rates — 5 percent mortality instead of 19 percent in major amputations. Later, when antibiotics came along, his prediction came true.

In addition to McKittrick, the Deaconess listed other eminent surgeons and physicians from Boston's leading teaching hospitals on its staff: urologists Harvard Crabtree and George Gilbert Smith, gynecologist Joe Vincent Meigs, general and thoracic surgeon Richard H. Sweet, oral and plastic surgeon Varaztad H. Kazanjian, neurosurgeon W. Jason Mixter, cancer surgeon Ernest Daland, cardiologist Burton E. Hamilton, and internists Joseph H. Aub and Earle Chapman. For many of these doctors, however, the Deaconess was an occasional convenience, not an institution to which they were deeply committed. Their ties to other hospitals, usually Massachusetts General, but also Peter Bent Brigham or Boston City, ran much deeper.

There were, however, independent practitioners on the staff who did use the Deaconess as a primary hospital. Internist Theodore

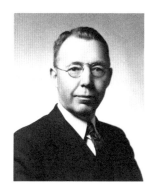

DR. LELAND S. MCKITTRICK, CA. 1940S. *A talented general surgeon, McKittrick received his early training in diabetic care with Daniel Fiske Jones and Elliott Joslin and became assistant to Jones in 1919, the day after completing his residency at Massachusetts General Hospital. McKittrick succeeded Jones as surgeon-in-chief of Palmer Hospital and was instrumental in focusing attention on the care of the diabetic foot. He was the first surgeon to receive the Banting Medal from the American Diabetic Association.*

Badger, who became a nationally recognized pulmonary specialist and taught at Massachusetts General Hospital, concentrated a good deal of his practice at the Deaconess. Gorham Brigham, whose huge practice and affluent patients gave him great influence in the hospital, was chief of medicine at *both* the Deaconess and Palmer Hospital from 1936 to 1946. He wielded immense power in deciding who would or would not be given staff privileges and he was never shy about exercising it.

Harry W. Goodall likewise had a large internal medicine practice, which included a number of wealthy patients, among them the presidents of five Boston banks. When Goodall died prematurely in 1935, Lyman H. Hoyt, who had been his assistant for six years, essentially inherited his practice. An Iowan who had been a track star at the University of Iowa, where he had also gone to medical school, Hoyt had great energy and vitality and a wonderful human touch. A master diagnostician and general internist, Hoyt became known for his devotion to patients and to New England Deaconess Hospital as well.

Nearly sixty years later, Hoyt recalled that in the 1930s and 1940s he had also been on the staff of Peter Bent Brigham Hospital where he had been in charge of thyroid and goiter patients, many of whom wanted Frank Lahey to perform their surgery. Since Brigham surgeons were not then doing thyroidectomies, quite a few of these patients, with Hoyt's help, would have the procedure performed by Lahey at the Deaconess. Looking back, Hoyt was amazed that he had not been expelled from the Brigham staff.

Among the other busy independent staff members who came to the Deaconess were Roger Graves, an outstanding urologist, Clifford Franseen, a superb technical surgeon and soft-spoken man whom many doctors used themselves, and Louisa Paine Tingley, a fair-minded and accomplished ophthalmologist, who performed numerous cataract operations. Lois Preston vividly recalled that Tingley drove an electric car and always wore a black skirt, a man-tailored shirt, and a necktie. Before examining each patient, Tingley would insist on having a fresh bar of soap to wash her hands.

THE LAHEY CLINIC

The Lahey Clinic, the third limb of the three-legged Deaconess stool, strengthened its reputation during the 1930s and 1940s because of its specialized surgery and medicine, excellent results, shrewd hiring practices, and attention to marketing. "Dr. Lahey's concept of a clinic practice was a team approach to patient care," wrote surgeon Herbert (Herb) Dan Adams. "His Clinic was not just the common version of group practice, a group of doctors banded together for their personal benefits, but group expertise concentrated for the best possible care and welfare of the patients — Group Patient Care! He carried this objective into the operating room as well. He expected and demanded smooth cooperation at all times from every member of his team and the O.R. personnel as well as perfect operating conditions — quiet, seriousness, good lighting, and excellent equipment."

At this time the Lahey Clinic had its own operating-room nurses and dominated certain operating rooms and surgical floors in the Deaconess Building, while the independent surgeons ruled the roost at Palmer — indeed there were two separate staffs in these years, one for the Deaconess and one for Palmer. There were no operating rooms in Baker. So separate were the two worlds that one memorable day Gorham Brigham was denied entry into a Deaconess operating room where one of his patients was undergoing surgery by a Lahey physician.

The Lahey Clinic did not confine itself to New England Deaconess Hospital, however, relying on New England Baptist Hospital at least as much. Two smaller hospitals, the Robert Breck Brigham and Corey Hill, were used for overflow, usually for less serious cases and less expensive accommodations. The Lahey Clinic also utilized certain other specialty facilities. Never one to lose a minute, Lahey himself was chauffeured in surgical garb from hospital to hospital in the back of a Cadillac.

Certain Lahey Clinic doctors did tend to concentrate their work in one or another hospital, however. For example, Sara Jordan, who achieved international recognition as a gastroenterologist, worked primarily at New England Baptist Hospital, where she cared for John F. Kennedy when he was a sickly young man. Reportedly, Jordan was able to exert greater influence over the Baptist's dietary department than she ever could at the Deaconess, where the food service was heavily focused on diabetics. Jordan was a particular favorite of Frank Lahey, who once told Herb Adams "she was the only woman I ever knew that acted like a woman but thought like a man."

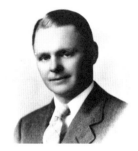

Dr. LYMAN H. HOYT, CA. 1942. *An internal medicine specialist, Hoyt served as physician-in-chief from 1956 to 1958. The hospital's medical teaching service was named in his honor. Beloved by his patients, Hoyt retired at the age of eighty-six after fifty-eight years in practice.*

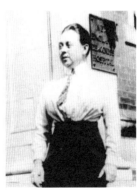

Dr. LOUISA PAINE TINGLEY, CA. 1920. *Ophthalmic surgeon Tingley worked as a private school teacher of German for ten years to save money for her medical education at Tufts Medical School.*

The Lahey Clinic's multispecialist approach was no longer in such a small minority. Group practices had begun to proliferate in the United States; by the early 1930s, there were approximately 150 private group clinics, with 1,500 to 2,000 doctors employed. In the midst of the Depression, such clinics offered doctors a greater degree of economic security and the opportunity to concentrate on their profession without having to worry about collecting fees. The Lahey Clinic paid its doctors' medical society dues and malpractice insurance, assisted them in producing scholarly articles, and encouraged them to speak at professional meetings, both of which helped spread the word about the clinic and attracted referrals.

Yet individual practitioners still disapproved of group practice. "Throughout the 1930s," historian Rosemary Stevens has written, "the AMA [American Medical Association] and its local societies waged war against group practice and other organized medical systems under the rubric of the 'corporate practice of medicine.' The AMA passed a resolution in 1934 requiring that medical staffs of hospitals accredited for internships include only members of the local medical society; doctors were expected to toe the party line."

Many doctors did not have to be coerced to embrace the official party line. Group practice ran counter to the way medicine had traditionally been practiced. It posed a threat to physician autonomy and seemed to introduce an impersonal and corporate element that made many doctors uncomfortable. In the view of some physicians, working on a salary as employees of a clinic seemed unethical, possibly entailing a violation of the Hippocratic oath — only a short step away from socialized medicine, therefore threatening not only individual doctors' autonomy, but potentially the amount of money they might be able to earn. Yet Lahey himself was politically conservative and an outspoken opponent of group health insurance plans, of socialized medicine, and of turning medicine into a commodity. A member of the American Medical Association's old guard, Lahey served as that organization's president from 1941 to 1942.

Herb Adams, who had been a chief resident at Massachusetts General and was later asked by Daniel Fiske Jones to be his assistant, recalled Jones's reaction when in 1936 Adams told of his plan to take a job with the Lahey Clinic instead. Jones "never liked Dr. Lahey," Adams recounted, "and on numerous occasions had expressed his dislike in no uncertain terms. . . .

With much foot dragging and real terror in my heart, I finally faced him in his office and received in navy terms a real 'dressing down.' In a very bitter and resentful tirade, he told me I was making the biggest mistake of my life!" Fortunately, it did not turn out that way; except for time out for military service, Adams spent a fulfilling career at the Lahey Clinic, eventually becoming its director.

Lahey business manager Linda Strand and a group of specially trained "pricers" implemented Lahey's sliding-fee scale. Clinic doctors never became involved in either setting fees or collecting them. Patients paid according to their financial status and ability. The poor, who paid no fees, constituted about 10 percent of those accepted as patients. They of course had to have a condition in which the clinic had special expertise. Most patients paid an intermediate fee, but the clinic would arrange time payments. There was no limit to what the affluent were charged, though there was some bargaining at this level. The Lahey Clinic attracted prominent and wealthy patients from throughout America and abroad.

IN 1936 WHEN HERB ADAMS JOINED THE LAHEY CLINIC, there were three acknowledged senior surgeons on its staff: Lahey, Richard B. Cattell, and Samuel Marshall, who specialized respectively in thyroid, biliary, and gastro-intestinal surgery, though all were general surgeons and never strictly confined themselves to one area. Cattell was a master technician and an extraordinarily fast and prodigious worker. He probably surpassed Lahey himself, who had been his preceptor, in sheer technical virtuosity, speed, and volume of work. According to Adams and other observers, Marshall, an excellent surgeon but an insecure person, envied and resented Cattell and sought to undermine him with Lahey. Trouble was already brewing over succession in the Lahey kingdom, though it would not reach a crisis until the 1950s.

Younger Lahey surgeons in the 1930s and 1940s also included Reeve Betts, Bentley Colcock, Richard H. Overholt, and Neil Swinton. Typically, they had come to the clinic as Lahey Fellows, a kind of preceptor-ship which also served as a testing ground for possible appointments to staff positions. This training program stood completely independent of Harvard or any other medical school. And although Lahey had once been a professor simultaneously at Harvard and Tufts, he had become disillusioned with academic medicine, keeping his distance and not allowing his staff to accept

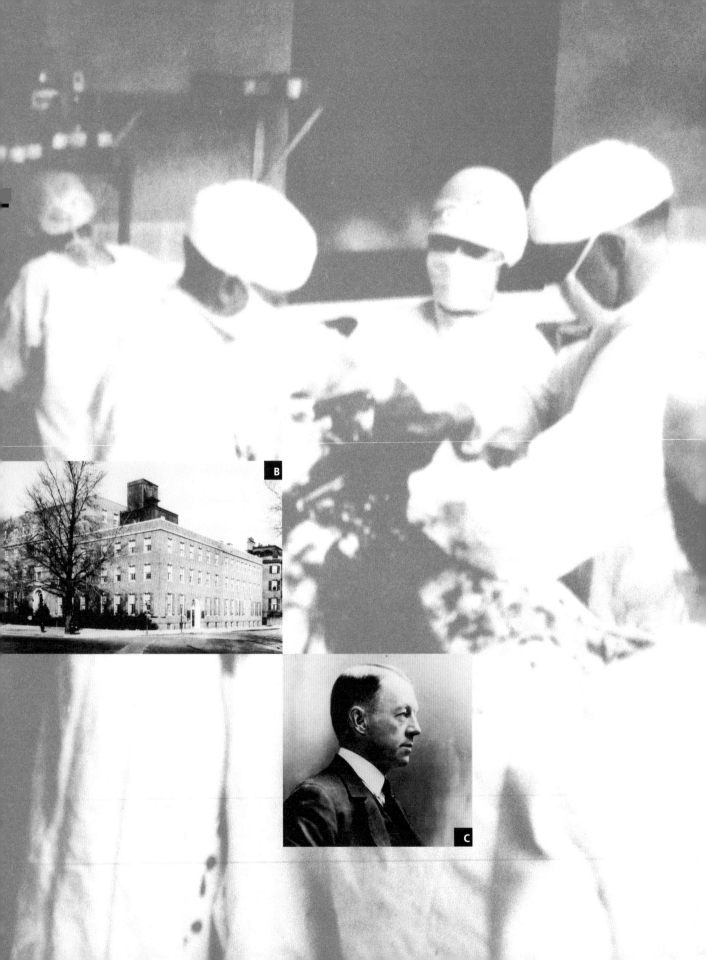

academic appointments. Many academically based doctors, on the other hand, shared the general medical view of clinics as an invidious form of "corporate medicine."

In the early 1930s, Lahey also developed a neurosurgery specialty within the clinic, hiring Gilbert Horrax to lead it. Horrax had spent many years at Peter Bent Brigham Hospital assisting Harvey Cushing, the legendary father of neurosurgery in this country. Horrax moved to the Deaconess following Cushing's retirement in 1932. A thorough gentleman and a methodical surgeon, Horrax was joined in the late 1930s by James L. Poppen, who, after a career in professional baseball, had received his surgical training in Chicago.

An extraordinarily deft and fast surgeon, Poppen was, according to Lahey neurosurgeon Charles Fager, "aggressive, dynamic, an absolute genius." Poppen achieved certain results in the operating room that have not been equaled since, observed Fager, a recognized master himself. Poppen also possessed the uncommon attribute of being very modest about his own accomplishments and abilities. Horrax and Poppen had patients with brain tumors referred to them from throughout New England, and the Deaconess, which had a special group of highly trained neurosurgical nurses, probably had the region's busiest neurosurgical service in the 1930s and 1940s, inheriting an area that formerly had been the territory of Harvey Cushing alone. By 1948, Lahey neurosurgeons had removed more than 1,400 brain tumors.

Richard Overholt was another notable young surgeon who joined the Lahey Clinic in the early 1930s. Overholt had grown up in a small town in Nebraska, the son of strict Methodist schoolteachers. After attending teachers' college in his hometown, Overholt got a job as principal of a small school, where he also taught and coached. While teaching, he boarded with a local physician, discovered *Gray's Anatomy,* and then began, at the doctor's invitation, to accompany him on house calls. Within a year, Overholt enrolled at the University of Nebraska Medical School.

During his first year of medical school, Overholt was hit by a car. His hospital roommate was a young boy who had become seriously ill from a lung abscess caused by aspirating a piece of food. As Overholt's own condition steadily improved, he watched the youngster's worsen

A A RARE PHOTOGRAPH OF DR. FRANK H. LAHEY IN SURGERY *(right) in the Deaconess Hospital operating room, ca. 1926. An internationally recognized surgeon, Lahey was one of the hospital's busiest doctors. His practice helped to fill Deaconess surgical rooms as he performed intricate procedures on the thyroid and the biliary and gastrointestinal tracts. Upon his death Dr. Claude Hunt wrote in the* American Journal of Surgery, *"He stood as a giant in the field of surgery . . . . There was something within him that could not and would not be deterred."*

B HOME OF THE LAHEY CLINIC *on Commonwealth Avenue in Boston, 1945.*

C DR. LAHEY, CA. 1936.

horribly, until he was wheeled out to die in another part of the hospital. Overholt suspected that the boy would have been saved if the infected lung could have been removed or the pus drained. Thus began his lifelong interest in lung disease and illnesses of the chest.

Lahey discovered Overholt in 1931 at the University of Pennsylvania Hospital where the latter had gone for his surgical training. Overholt joined the Lahey Clinic the next year as a general surgeon, but stipulated that he be free to pursue his interest in thoracic surgery, a field that was still in its infancy. Indeed, only three physicians were doing thoracic surgery in Boston and their work was part time. Overholt took a particular interest in tuberculosis patients, who had largely been ignored by surgeons. He performed thoracoplasties (surgical removal of ribs and collapsing of chest wall as curative procedure) on ten patients from the Norfolk Sanitarium. Since all ten survived and nine returned to a normal life, he was soon flooded with requests for the procedure and organized "saddle-back" teams to sanatoria throughout Massachusetts and Rhode Island.

Overholt's experience with chest-wall surgery prepared him for the next step, open-chest surgery. After performing three successful lobectomies, he was ready to attempt what had previously been tried elsewhere in the world, but had rarely succeeded — a pneumonectomy, total removal of a lung. In 1933 Overholt attended the annual meeting of thoracic surgeons where he was encouraged to hear E. A. Graham's account of the successful left pneumonectomy he had recently performed in St. Louis. In November of that year, at Deaconess Hospital, the thirty-two-year-old Overholt performed the world's first right pneumonectomy on a thirty-three-year-old woman. The patient survived the procedure and lived another twenty-nine years. Details of the operation were subsequently reported in the *Journal of Thoracic Surgery.*

Overholt was a pioneer in public health as well. Clinical and anatomical observations led him to conclude that smoking damaged people's health, and he began to speak out on the dangers of smoking in the 1930s, decades before such a stance was accepted by the surgical and medical worlds, not to mention the broader community.

Eager to devote his time completely to thoracic surgery, Overholt left the Lahey Clinic in 1938, taking Reeve Betts with him and setting up the Overholt Thoracic Clinic on Beacon Street in Boston. Lahey had been skeptical about the economic viability of thoracic surgery, since the largest volume of likely candidates for such surgery tended to be poor and were in state-operated tuberculosis sanatoria. Overholt was never wont of referrals, however. He was also entrepreneurial and clever about how to make a good living in his chosen specialty. He eventually won contracts to care for patients at public and private sanatoria throughout eastern Massachusetts, New Hampshire, and Rhode Island. Much of the work was done locally, but more difficult operations were brought to the Deaconess, where Overholt had an isolation ward on the fourth floor of the Deaconess Building. Through the years Overholt developed new techniques in thoracic surgery, published a standard text, *The Techniques of Pulmonary Resection,* in 1948, and hired additional surgeons to work with him.

INCLUDED IN LAHEY'S VISION of a group approach to patient care was his support for a fairly new medical specialty, anesthesiology. Lahey was an early enthusiast of physician-anesthetists although in the Palmer operating rooms, Jones and McKittrick usually worked with free-lance nurse anesthetists from Massachusetts General. Lincoln F. Sise had begun to specialize in anesthesia soon after his graduation from Harvard Medical School in 1901. He joined the Lahey Clinic at its inception and served as its chief anesthetist until his retirement in 1939. Before he left, he had been joined by Philip D. Woodbridge and Urban H. Eversole, who trained at the Mayo Clinic and the University of Wisconsin, respectively, both early centers of physician training in anesthesia.

   The Lahey Clinic itself became a leader in anesthesia training and started a program for physician-anesthetists; in the 1930s there were only four other accredited curricula for physician training in anesthesia in the United States. "There were four of us residents — we always worked under the constant supervision of a senior man — in the O.R. — not in his office, library, or at home," recalled Morris J. Nicholson, who started his residency in 1938. Beginning in 1936, the Lahey Clinic gradually hired four additional staff members who were products of its own anesthesia training program, Joseph Crehan, Leo V. Hand, Nicholson, and Robert Orr. Hand left Lahey in 1946, going into private practice and crossing the Rubicon to serve the independent surgeons in Palmer. He was joined two years later by Francis Audin, who had also trained at the clinic before moving to Philadelphia.

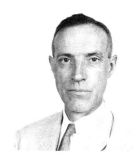

DR. GILBERT HORRAX, CA. 1956. *Closely associated with the father of American neurosurgery, Dr. Harvey Cushing, Horrax founded the Lahey Clinic's Department of Neurosurgery in 1932. The hospital library was dedicated in his honor in 1959.*

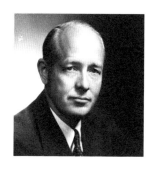

DR. RICHARD H. OVERHOLT, CA. 1950. *A skilled cardiothoracic surgeon, Overholt performed the world's first right pneumonectomy at the Deaconess in 1933. A pioneer in fighting the ravages of cigarette smoking, Overholt lectured widely on the deleterious effects of smoking.*

SERVING THE THREE-LEGGED STOOL

Despite the tripartite nature of the Deaconess, certain services were shared by all three components. Two hospital-based specialties, roentgenology and pathology, served the independent staff, the Joslin doctors, and the Lahey Clinic alike. At first, the hospital had difficulty filling the gap left by Lawrie Morrison's death in 1933, unsuccessfully offering the job to several roentgenologists before Joseph H. Marks became head of the service in 1937, assisted by Isabel K. Bogan and Hugh F. Hare. Apparently the radiology staff derived most of their incomes as hospital employees, the rest as private physicians. Because X-ray equipment was so expensive, this specialty virtually had to be hospital-based — in 1935 the Deaconess paid $20,000 for a 400,000-volt machine for deep radiotherapy manufactured by General Electric, which was installed in Palmer. As with radium and radon therapy, the effects and effectiveness of radiotherapy were ill understood at the time, but the treatment proved popular. By 1939, more than 3,000 radiotherapy treatments were given in Palmer and two years later, over 5,000.

Precise and a stickler for detail, Marks kept his subordinates on a short leash, even keeping track of their hours of arrival and departure. He was insistent, demanding, and cross. "Your place is certainly the crossroads of the hospital and I mean cross," kidded Bob Brownlee, who greatly admired Marks. He was immensely compassionate toward patients, however, and doctors appreciated the high quality of the services he provided. In 1944, the Deaconess, Peter Bent Brigham, and Children's hospitals combined to offer a residency in roentgenology, leading to certification by the American Board of Radiology. "It is our belief," wrote Marks, "that such a combined service will be of greater value to the resident than would a similar period of time spent in any one of the three hospitals." This residency was a forerunner of future collaborations in radiological science among area hospitals.

The pathology department, meanwhile, flourished under Shields Warren's leadership, providing excellent laboratory service not only to the Deaconess, but to the Baptist, Pondville, Huntington Memorial (until it was closed and relocated to Massachusetts General in the early 1940s), and a changing roster of other hospitals as well. Pondville, the first state-operated cancer hospital in America, had opened its doors in 1927 and eventually supplanted Palmer Hospital as the place where poor patients were apt to seek cancer treatment. (Massachusetts joined New York as a leader in publicly supported treatment to fight cancer.) In addition, Warren and his colleagues consulted to a widening circle of hospitals. For many years, the state's tumor diagnosis service was based in the department and was overseen by Olive Gates, an excellent pathologist, who spent her entire career at the Deaconess and was a key Warren collaborator.

These additional services brought extra income into the department, which Warren used to dole out to supplement his staff's meager base salaries and to support research and training. Like Joslin and Lahey, Warren was the lord and master of his own bailiwick, so there was nothing unusual or untoward about these practices.

As department head, Warren was intolerant of errors; those who committed them were typically asked to leave. Indeed, his enthusiasm for his work was legendary and a steady stream of residents came to train under him. Typically, four or five new residents or fellows came each year before the war, when the length of a pathology residency was not yet established. According to Tillman McDaniel, Warren had a vacation home on Cape Cod where residents were often invited guests. Residents were not always fond of Warren's cordiality, however, because he would expect them to haul rocks to build up his pier. Yet Warren was also known as a kind, considerate, and warm individual, and completely honest.

Often residents were supported by research grants of one kind or another. William A. Meissner, Warren's successor in pathology, for example, came as a Littauer Fellow in 1942, a cancer fellowship granted by Harvard that was actually based at Huntington Memorial Hospital. His salary was $2,000 a year, but about three weeks after his arrival at the Deaconess, Warren's assistant suddenly quit and Meissner was asked to succeed him — and with the appointment came a $400 increase.

The pathology laboratory conducted many clinical tests — 165,558 in 1940. This number grew after the introduction of sulfanila mides and it expanded even further after the advent of antibiotics. The volume of bacteriological examinations increased from 1,622 in 1935 to 3,960 in 1940, which led to the hiring of the hospital's first bacteriologist. Warren also oversaw the hospital's blood bank (established in 1942), its solution room, and electrocardiography, all of which were growing in importance. In 1944, Deaconess pathologists performed 6,381 surgical

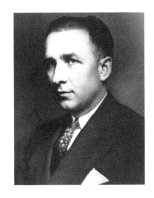

Dr. Joseph H. Marks, ca. 1931. As the head of roentgenology and successor to Laurie Morrison, Marks joined the Deaconess staff in 1937. In his first year the department performed 5,594 diagnostic exams and 4,198 X-ray treatments. A graduate of Harvard Medical School, Marks oversaw the rapid growth in X-ray technology that occurred in the decades following World War II. In later years he pursued his special interest in radiation therapy.

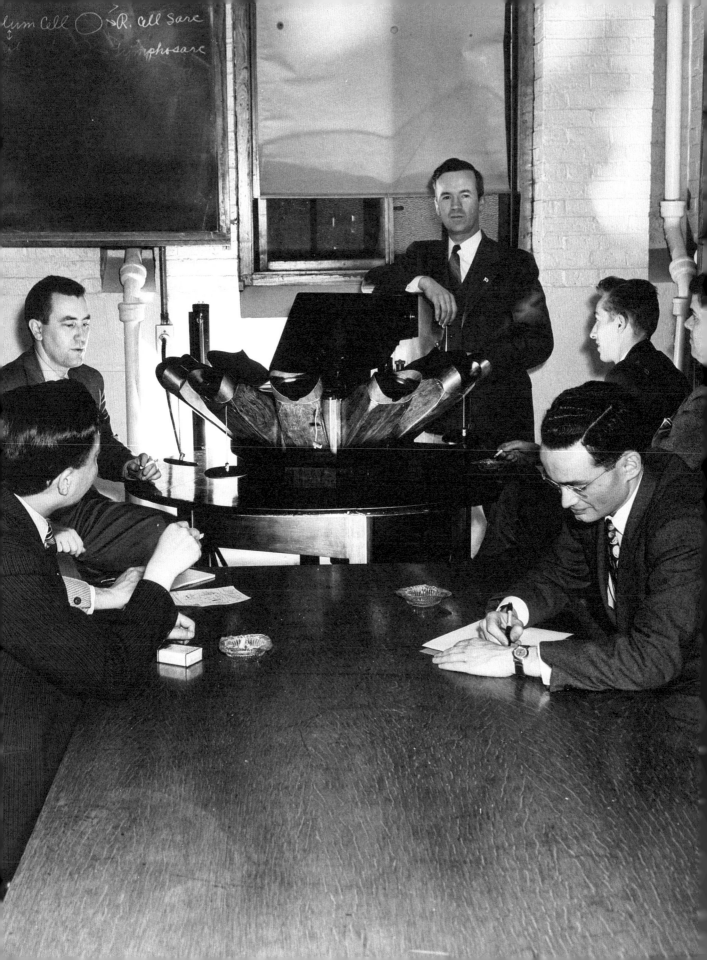

examinations and 171 autopsies. An invaluable learning tool for doctors, autopsies were typically performed on approximately half of all hospital mortalities. At the Deaconess a special signal would ring when an autopsy was about to begin so that interested doctors could attend.

Warren and his colleagues were involved in anatomic as well as clinical pathology. Warren conducted research on stomach cancer and leukemia and world-renowned research on the pathology of radiation reaction. He also explored the diagnostic possibilities of radioisotopes, an area where he himself came to feel he made his most important scientific contribution. He continued to work on diabetes mellitus and in 1938 published a revised edition of his book on that subject. The laboratory conducted some animal research, but space constraints restricted its activity. Work was also restricted by a lack of endowment; research was primarily supported by foundation grants.

ROOM TO GROW

In the late 1930s the Deaconess was bulging at the seams. "Every department of the Hospital is handicapped by the lack of room," Warren Cook wrote in the 1937 report. He also proposed a solution — a new structure to be located between the Deaconess and Baker buildings which "would allow us to centralize administration, laboratories, X-ray, record rooms, kitchen stores, etc. Here we could also build a new operating suite and add sufficient beds to allow us to separate our services adequately." Cook insisted, "This is not just a dream. This should be seriously considered." It was. In 1938 the Executive Committee appointed a seven-member planning committee, which included Frank Lahey, and hired architects Coolidge Shepley Bulfinch and Abbott to begin working on preliminary plans.

In the ensuing years, Cook crusaded publicly for the new Central Building. In the 1938 annual report he highlighted the efficiencies that could be gained. "We have three cashiers' offices, three admitting offices, two record rooms, two X-ray plants, three laboratories, and a half dozen receiving points," he wrote. "You can readily see the savings we could make if we centralized these services in a new building."

DR. WILLIAM A. MEISSNER AND PATHOLOGY RESIDENTS AND FELLOWS, LATE 1940S. *Pictured leading a microscopic slide conference, Meissner used a new and exciting "Scopicon," which allowed projection of a microscopic slide inside the box. The image could then be viewed through six "portholes." The Scopicon was so large and cumbersome that it could not be accommodated in pathology and was set up in an abandoned storeroom in the basement of the Palmer Building.*

Crowding only worsened with time. "Each year we feel that we cannot take more patients, yet our statistics this year show that our patient days reached 103,445 which is 849 more than the figure for 1939," Cook reported in 1940. "During the year we averaged over 200 patients daily waiting admission, and the average daily number of patients in the house ran above 92 percent. The facts are simply that we cannot accommodate the demand for patients from our Staff with our present bed capacity and I see no relief for this situation except expansion."

Pressure from the Lahey Clinic for additional beds and operating capacity was particularly strong. During this period, Lahey surgeons began to operate in two shifts at the Deaconess, morning and afternoon. Lahey himself became a frequent visitor to Cook's office to plead for more hospital beds and more operating rooms. In early 1939, Cook presented a letter to the Executive Committee from Lahey "inquiring as to the possibilities of having the use of some beds at the Palmer," something which McKittrick and the independent staff undoubtedly must have resisted.

In November 1939, Cook spoke to the Executive Committee about the possibility of a new building, or, at the very least, the erection of a new operating suite atop the Deaconess Building. Four months later, the Executive Committee recommended launching a capital campaign for the erection of a new building *and* an operating suite. A little over a year later, in May 1941, following extensive discussions with many groups and individuals, Cook spelled out to the trustees what he saw as the "only three alternatives": "(1) Raise the fund[s] and build the building and meet the growing hospital demand; (2) Build a modern operating suite and turn the hospital over to the clinics; (3) Remain as we are and limit the clinics still further with a possible resulting loss of the clinics." Unless the trustees were prepared to surrender the hospital to the clinics or risk the hospital's life without them, it is clear that they really had only one choice — the first.

Cook presented a letter from Joslin favoring that option. Cook also expressed his optimism about securing the necessary funds because of the hospital's illustrious personalities. With one dissenter, Henry S. Rogerson, the trustees adopted the Executive Committee's recommendation that a new five-story building be constructed and that a fund-raising firm be employed to assist in raising the necessary money. The trustees had evidently learned a lesson from their previous building projects — they endeavored to raise money in advance rather than borrowing.

THE HOSPITAL'S FINANCIAL PICTURE BRIGHTENED considerably in the late 1930s and still further in the early 1940s due to a number of developments. First was the Deaconess's sheer volume of activity — it operated at 90 percent capacity year after year. By comparison, the typical Massachusetts hospital capacity in these years ran in the low 70s. Particularly busy areas with special capabilities and technologies, including pathology, operating rooms, radiology, and the pharmacy store, generated additional revenues. Second, the hospital was able to raise rates as costs escalated during and after the war. Collections also became more reliable and assured, partly because of improving economic conditions and better collection methods but also because of the advent of hospital insurance.

Blue Cross had begun to gain acceptance in the 1930s, particularly in states such as Massachusetts, where nonprofit hospitals predominated. Deaconess Hospital was pleased to participate in these plans as they came along, in part because they held out hope of keeping Washington at bay. In 1943, three influential congressional Democrats proposed expanding Social Security to create a comprehensive, prepaid medical-care system, a cause which President Harry Truman later adopted in his successful whistle-stop campaign of 1948. "Blue Cross is another effort to save the voluntary hospitals of America from federal control," is what Cook bluntly asserted in 1949. Indeed, by 1947, approximately half of the Deaconess's patients were members of Blue Cross, although the hospital's administration also complained that it was losing money because of ceilings the association placed on ancillary charges.

During this time the hospital continued to provide free care to indigent patients, though, it would appear, proportionately less than in the early decades. In the immediate postwar years, approximately six cents of the expense dollar went to free treatment, which was evidently covered by legacies limited to that purpose and supplemented by income from some unre-stricted bequests. In addition, the hospital's social service department, Warren Cook reported in 1943, brought in "approximately $25,000 annually from cities and towns on the bills of welfare patients." Two years later, social service director Gertrude Jameson reported that $28,000 had been received from "135 private and Public Welfare Departments."

Finally, bequests helped support the hospital's improving fiscal health. For example, in February 1939, New England Deaconess Hospital and the New England Deaconess Association reached a settlement in a legal

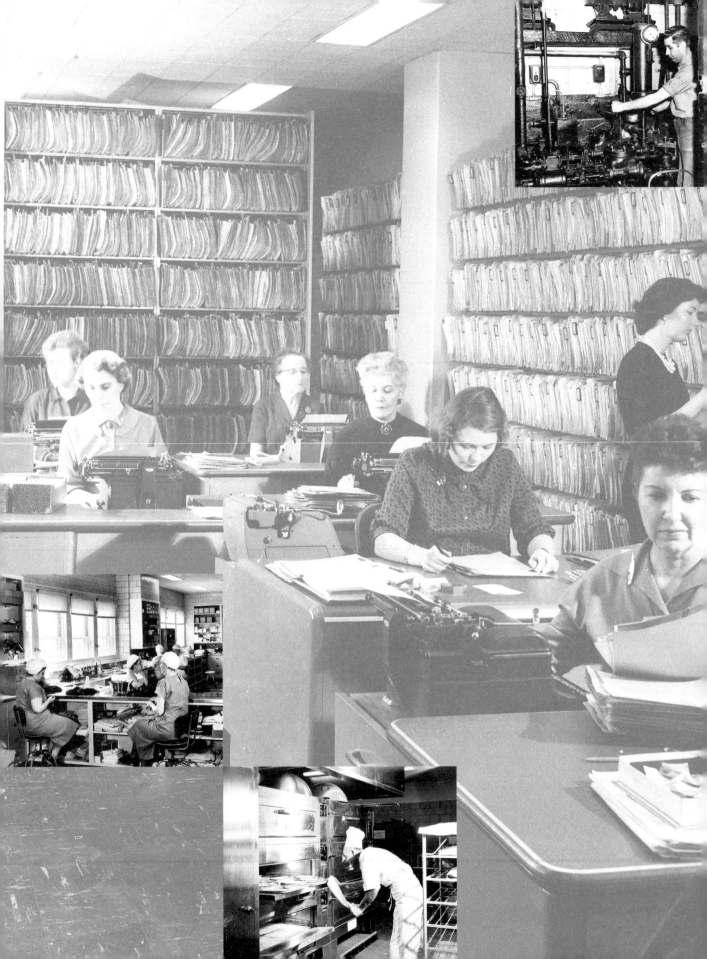

controversy involving the William A. Sargent estate. In 1938, while the case was still in court, the hospital was required to pay not only interest but principal on its mortgage with the John Hancock Mutual Insurance Company, amounting to more than $76,000. The hospital's total operating budget that year approached a million dollars. Having to pay that much per year had forced the hospital to curtail expenditures, so the settlement came as a great relief. Under the decision, the hospital could anticipate receiving $25,500 a year between 1940 and 1953 to be applied to paying off the John Hancock mortgage. The settlement included the following provision: "The Hospital will have Methodists constitute a majority of the members of its corporation after June 30, 1953 or after the John Hancock mortgage is paid if it should be paid sooner." (New corporation bylaws adopted in 1946 likewise required that a majority of the corporation be members of the Methodist Episcopal Church.) Other bequests were made in these years as well. In the ten years between 1937 and 1946, the hospital received close to $973,000, 80 percent of it unrestricted. By early 1945, the hospital's debt was reduced to $230,000. "I well remember when it stood at over a million and a quarter dollars," Cook commented with relief in the 1944 report.

Given the hospital's improving financial picture and the clear need for a new central building, it made perfect sense for the trustees to proceed with the capital campaign. Unfortunately, the timing was inauspicious. By 1941, hope was diminishing that the United States would be able to stay out of the conflict that had engulfed Europe and Asia. After the Japanese attacked Pearl Harbor on December 7, 1941, that hope vanished as the United States quickly declared war on Japan and Germany. The war effort placed a great strain on all hospitals, including the Deaconess, due to wartime shortages and because so many doctors and nurses went off to serve their country.

Although the war ended the Depression, it was hard to raise money in the midst of such uncertainty and distraction — many potential fund-raisers and donors were preoccupied with the war effort or in the service. It is therefore impressive that by September 1945, just after the war ended, the building fund actually had gathered $756,000 in cash and pledges. Yet building costs were beginning to rise and the original estimates of the building's expenses had escalated by 1944 from

STAFF OF DEACONESS HOSPITAL in the 1930s and 1940s. Despite the Depression and war, the hospital's staff and services grew to reflect the increasing complexity and sophistication of hospital care. Superintendent Warren Cook compared the hospital to a large hotel whose guests did not leave their beds. Service departments such as medical records, dietary, laundry, central processing, maintenance, and the pharmacy were busy hubs of activity.

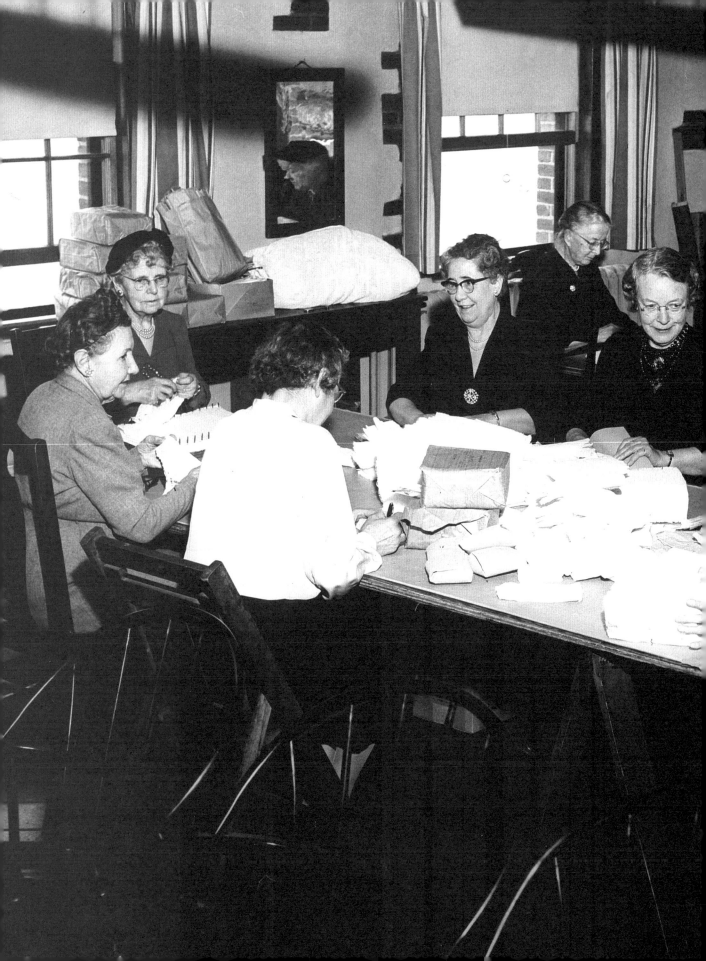

$1.5 to $1.8 million, a figure that included 200 new beds and an addition to Harris Hall. Moreover, manifestations of disharmony among medical staff within the hospital made it clear that Warren Cook's dream of combining expansion *and* centralization would not be easily achieved.

WARTIME SERVICE

DURING THE WAR, personnel shortages and turnover were the most serious problems that confronted the Deaconess and many other hospitals. By September 1942, for example, nearly half of the Lahey Clinic's doctors were in the service while the number of nurses at the Deaconess declined by 42 percent between September 1942 and September 1943. "The diminishing number of competent Hospital personnel of all kinds, doctors, nurses, technicians, skilled labor, as well as help for all departments of the Hospital, has been appalling," Warren Cook flatly stated in one report. "Four hundred and ninety-five (495) have come and gone during 1944."

Since the hospital census did not slacken during the war, it meant that those who did not join the armed services worked even harder than usual, nursing director Lois Preston has recalled. It also meant that promotions came quickly — Preston became a head nurse within three or four years of graduation. Some doctors and nurses either postponed or came out of retirement. Because of the shortage of doctors, nurses were allowed to give transfusions and intravenous solutions. The hospital administration was also given authority to commandeer private-duty nurses in urgent situations (with the permission of the patient's doctor).

To help secure workers and get professional advice on work-place efficiencies, the hospital's first personnel director was appointed in 1942, and a personnel department was established two years later under the direction of Ellen Adams (no relation to Herb). The nursing school, meanwhile, with some government assistance, expanded to meet heightened demand for nurses; in September 1944, the largest class in the school's history was enrolled. The school continued to admit two classes a year.

VOLUNTEERS ROLLING BANDAGES IN THE 1940S. *The volunteer surgical dressing assistants met every Wednesday morning to roll dressings from 1933 until 1960 when the hospital began to purchase ready-made dressings.*

THROUGHOUT THE WAR, volunteers played a vital role in filling staffing needs. In 1943, 1,251 individuals worked as volunteers in a variety of capacities, giving the equivalent of 4,700 eight-hour days. Many of the volunteers were new to the hospital, but quite a few came from the "Friends of the Deaconess," an organization which had begun as the Women's Association of New England Deaconess Hospital in 1931 to help raise money for new equipment and for charity patients. Many of the organization's members were doctors' wives, including Mrs. F. Gorham Brigham, Mrs. Shields Warren, Mrs. Howard Root, and Mrs. Leland McKittrick, though its founding president, Mrs. Alexander D. (Catherine) Grant, was not. She had become interested in helping the Deaconess after her son, a diabetic who had been near death in Children's Hospital, was transferred to the Deaconess. He became one of the first patients to receive insulin under Joslin's care. He thrived and continues to enjoy a long life, including his college years as a member of the Harvard football team.

In its first year, the Women's Association netted $201.15, a modest figure but one destined to grow. The group raised money in a variety of ways — by selling eggs and homemade food, through rummage sales and the establishment of a thrift shop, and, beginning in 1940, through Deaconess Hospital Night at the Boston Pops. The Association also engaged in volunteer work at the hospital, including regular meetings to make surgical dressings. In 1943, the Association became incorporated as the Friends of the Deaconess Hospital, Inc., a tax-exempt organization. "We feel justified in saying," Grant reported in 1944, "that the six volunteers who have given the most hours (Gray Ladies, Ward Aides, and Nurse's Aides) are all members of the Friends of the Deaconess. A large proportion of our group is beyond the age for strenuous ward jobs, but still continues faithfully to work twice a week on surgical dressings." For her own 4,300 hours as a Nurse's Aide, Grant received a special citation signed by President Roosevelt and the head of the American Red Cross.

ALTHOUGH MANY DEACONESS PERSONNEL performed military service, two of its doctors, Frank Lahey and Shields Warren, held particularly important positions in Washington. Lahey, who had served in World War I, did not go back into uniform, but became a weekly commuter to Washington early in the war and sometimes traveled abroad in an official capacity. He served as chief consultant to Admiral Ross McIntyre, the surgeon general of the navy, in which capacity he was brought in to examine President Franklin D. Roosevelt at the Bethesda Naval Hospital in 1944, ten months before Roosevelt's death.

Lahey's much more demanding task, however, came as chairman of the Procurement and Requirement Board, Selective Service for Physicians. The group was responsible for the selection and induction of doctors, balancing military needs against civilian ones, making sure that overzealous recruitment did not strip parts of the country of essential coverage. Herb Adams later observed that the only time he ever saw Lahey "depressed or frustrated in the slightest was on his return from some of his weekly visits to Washington during those early war years." Adams recalled, "He put his exceptionally keen mind and boundless drive and energy into the solution of complex manpower problems only to see them frequently undermined and bypassed by bureaucrats and special interests. In his dealings with the many problems of the Clinic and hospitals, he was used to having his decisions honored and carried out promptly and to the letter!"

Warren, meanwhile, became a naval officer and donned a uniform, but actually divided his time between the hospital and Washington, where his expertise in the safe handling of radioactivity was in great demand. He spent the latter part of 1945 on a special mission to Japan to study the effects of the atomic bomb. His investigations in Nagasaki and Hiroshima led to the establishment of the Atomic Bomb Casualty Commission, which studied the health consequences of radiation, and whose sponsorship was eventually assumed by the Japanese. After the war, Warren studied the medical problems arising from atomic bomb tests in the Bikini Islands and in 1948, he became the first director of the Division of Biology and Medicine at the Atomic Energy Commission.

During Warren's absences, Bill Meissner, a superb administrator, scientist, and gentleman, assumed day-to-day responsibility for the pathology lab, except for the time when he himself served on a hospital ship. Warren, however, remained chief pathologist. In 1948 he was appointed a full professor at Harvard Medical School under the title "Professor of Pathology at the New England Deaconess Hospital," with

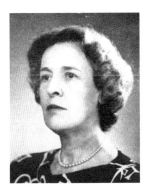

CATHERINE DELANO GRANT, CA. 1945. *One of the founders and the first president of the hospital's women's committee, Catherine Grant was a familiar face at the Deaconess for two decades. In 1943 the women's group incorporated as the Friends of the Deaconess Hospital, Inc. The group's first bequest was $10 to decorate patients' trays at Christmas. Over the years the Friends have provided important contributions of time and money to benefit the hospital and its patients.*

a portion of his salary paid by Harvard. Warren was the first and for many years the only Deaconess staff member to hold such a regular academic appointment, although many hospital staff members had previously held clinical appointments at Harvard, or at Tufts or Boston University.

During the war, the army and navy sent doctors to the Deaconess, sometimes by way of the Lahey Clinic, for training tours of three to six months. Young military doctors received experience in pathology, medicine, surgery, anesthesia, and radiology. Technicians also received training in radiology and in the hospital's laboratories.

POLITICAL TUG-OF-WAR

While a world war was being waged in Europe and the Pacific, a political tug-of-war was going on at the Deaconess over the proposed new Central Building. The three doctors' groups within the hospital, Lahey, Joslin, and the independents, were at odds over a number of basic questions. In the meantime, the hospital's trustees and administration were working to broker agreements and achieve consensus among the factions while simultaneously trying to uphold the hospital's own well-being. The number of unanswered questions was legion. How many beds and operating rooms would be available to each group? To what extent would groups control their own separate areas within the hospital? Who would be responsible for raising what part of the necessary funds? How did each group balance its own needs and aspirations against those of Deaconess Hospital as a whole?

None of those directly involved in debating these questions is alive to discuss them, but minutes of the Executive Committee and trustee meetings from the mid- and late 1940's hint at significant differences of opinion and at an atmosphere that was sometimes marked by suspicion. At a special meeting of the Board of Trustees on May 1, 1944, for example, Joslin asked that before passing the resolution authorizing the capital campaign, "the Trustees ratify the vote of the Staff setting up the principle of division of beds in the Hospital in accordance with the existing ratio, so that not over 40 percent of the beds would be allotted to any one group. After considerable discussion, Dr. Lahey stated that he did not wish to express his opinion with regard to this until after he had had a chance to consult with New England Baptist Hospital."

A month later, Cook wrote Lahey to confirm an understanding they had reached over the telephone. If Deaconess Hospital were to proceed with a campaign for $1.5 million to erect a new building of approximately 200 new beds, a new operating suite, and all necessary services, the hospital would need to have the Lahey Clinic's complete cooperation in raising the money "with the further understanding that the Lahey Clinic is to have a segregated [separate] unit of approximately 200 beds as well as a segregated [separate] operating suite, all of which has been agreed upon by the Staff of the Hospital and the Executive Committee of the Trustees."

Well after the capital campaign was under way, Lahey, who had been helping to raise money, embarked on an another fundraising drive, for a new pavilion at New England Baptist Hospital. This naturally caused concern among the trustees. Even more of a problem, however, was created by Joslin's attempt in 1946 to alter the Deaconess building program to incorporate a separate structure completely dedicated to diabetic care and research. For this purpose, Joslin had already created a separate Diabetic Fund, with representatives from Harvard and Tufts medical schools. He explained to Stanley MacMullen, chairman of the Deaconess Executive Committee, that he had done so because "in recent years we have been informed by certain influential donors who might well give one or more hundred thousand dollars that they were averse to contributing to any sectarian institution or even to the Deaconess."

The trustees offered to give Joslin the space he wanted in the new Central Building, but opposed a separate facility on practical grounds. For one thing, almost a million dollars had already been raised for the agreed-upon plan. If Joslin insisted on a separate structure, the trustees offered to give him $200,000 toward it, a little more than their records indicated he had raised toward the Central Building. Joslin was not satisfied with this solution, however; nor would he abandon his idea of a separate facility.

In September of 1946 the issue was debated at a special meeting of the trustees. Joslin made his case and was backed by Catherine Grant, who made a motion to approve Joslin's objective. MacMullen and William B. Snow, president of the Suffolk Savings Bank and chairman of the building fund drive, spoke against the motion, and so did Lahey, who "said that decentralizing was unwise, that the hospital had made a mistake in the past by decentralizing some of its activities and that the mistake should not be made again." Lahey "also said that possibly it would be unjust to the others if the original plan were abandoned or radically changed at this time." The motion was defeated.

The following spring, both the independent staff and the Joslin group successfully objected to Lahey's request that his clinic be given 40 percent of the *total* beds in the hospital and that such beds be allocated in one block. The existing agreement provided that the Lahey Clinic receive no more than 40 percent of the *available* beds. Don Lowry, whose difficult job it was to assign beds, explained that under the existing arrangement, he was able to give from 106 to 110 to the Lahey Clinic, approximately 40 percent of a 90 percent occupancy. If Lahey's request were implemented, Gorham Brigham asserted, there would be insufficient beds for the general staff, since it would effectively give an additional twenty spaces to Lahey. Brigham also argued that many Lahey doctors were there for training purposes only and would not remain as practitioners in Massachusetts.

Nevertheless, despite the ongoing turf battle, the capital campaign and expansion plans went forward. In 1947, the hospital successfully petitioned the city for the discontinuance of Deaconess Road as a public way and then bought a section of the street where the Central Building would rise. That year, too, the trustees doubled the fund-raising target, to $3 million. They also approved a construction loan of up to $1 million, to be secured by a mortgage on all the hospital's real property, except the George F. Baker Clinic Building. In addition, they rescinded the policy they had adopted in 1938 requiring a dollar-for-dollar endowment fund to support the operation of any new building.

It is not hard to understand why the trustees were willing to move ahead, indeed, why it was practical that they do so. The pie was being expanded, so all three doctors' groups would be getting more. The Depression and war were over and so was the accompanying gloom. The hospital's own finances were sound and prospects were excellent — old debt had now been retired; the hospital was operating at or above capacity; rates were able to be raised in line with cost increases; Blue Cross insurance promised a reliable stream of reimbursements; the hospital's independent staff and clinics were thriving; and its patients were pleased with the care.

As the building fund continued to raise money in the late 1940s, certain other changes were in the air. In 1946, Howard Root succeeded Brigham as physician-in-chief in the Deaconess division and the following year Richard Cattell followed Lahey as surgeon-in-chief. Both Brigham and Lahey stepped down voluntarily because of advancing age, though each would continue to be an important presence, as would Joslin. It was a definite sign, however, of an inevitable evolution in the hospital's long-standing central cast of characters.

With the end of the war and the beginning of a postwar rush of activity, academic medicine and scientific research were beginning to loom larger in the hospital's future. Warren's appointment to an academic professorship at Harvard was one clear manifestation of this. Warren was also instrumental in securing a $400,000 grant from the U.S. Public Health Service to build a new cancer institute with both laboratory space and a cancer detection clinic. The sizable funding for this project reflected two growing national developments: the emergence of the federal government as a source of research funds and the increasing attention to cancer as a targeted disease. (Into the 1930s, cancer was not considered a smart thing for young scientists to study because no progress had been made. "If a great scientist at the end of a brilliant career wants to make a fool of himself, he takes up the problem of cancer," a medical historian sardonically observed.)

In June of 1950 ground was broken for the new cancer center. The hospital's medical staff, in the largest meeting that it had ever held, had approved this initiative in 1948. In reporting to the Executive Committee, Howard Root also "discussed the closer relationship that may ultimately exist with the Harvard Medical group and the group of hospitals in our neighborhood." The minutes do not indicate what the staff's reaction to such a relationship was on that particular day, but in light of what was to follow, one might assume that they did not greet this prospect with unmitigated joy.

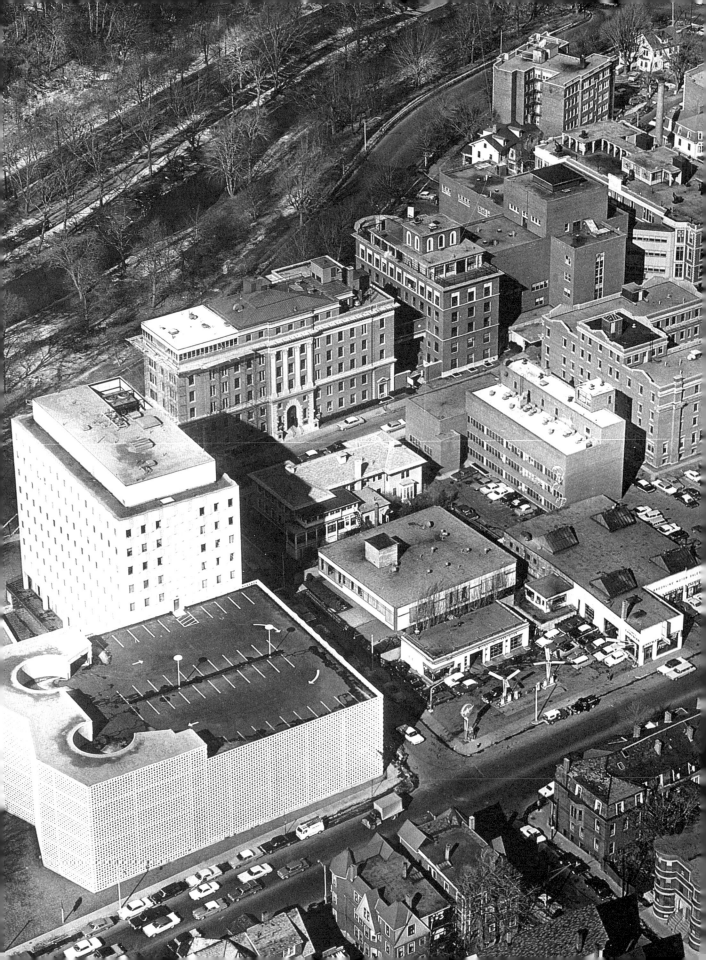

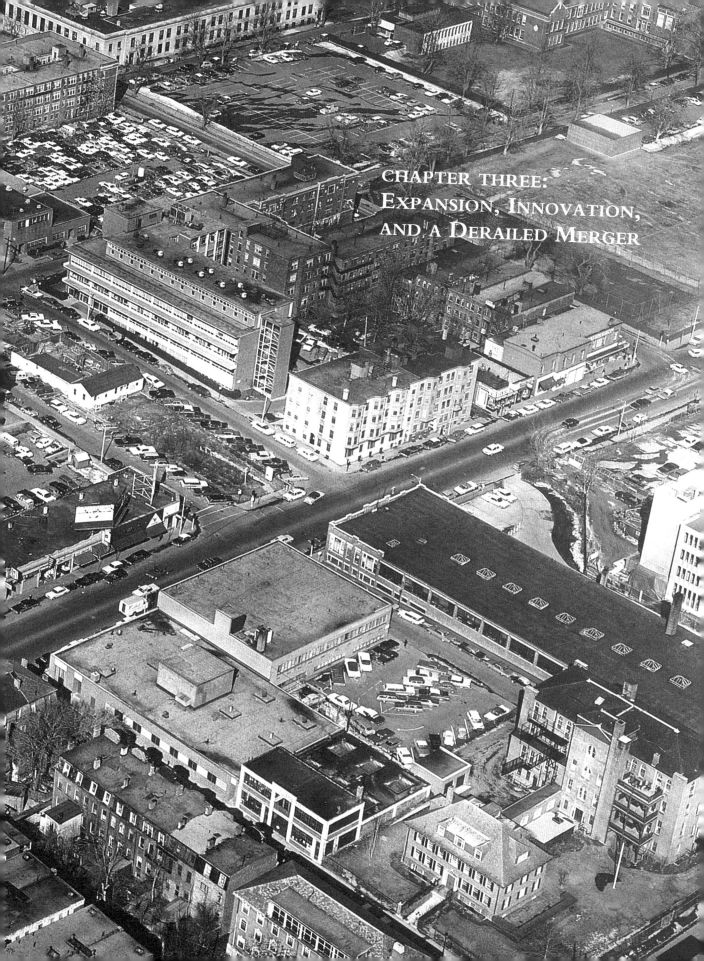

CHAPTER THREE:
EXPANSION, INNOVATION,
AND A DERAILED MERGER

Overleaf:

*Aerial photograph of the
Deaconess Hospital "complex,"
ca. 1965, captures the
enormous physical growth of
the Deaconess and other
institutions in the Longwood
medical area. Vestiges of an
earlier era still remain, however,
in the groupings of three-
and four-story apartment
buildings, ground-level parking
lots, and even single-family
homes. In time nearly all of the
remaining real estate would be
purchased by the growing
medical institutions for clinical,
research, and administrative
needs.*

CHAPTER THREE:
EXPANSION, INNOVATION,
AND A DERAILED MERGER

For the next two decades, from the early 1950s into the early 1970s, New England Deaconess Hospital expanded significantly, both in terms of physical plant and services provided. During this time, a new generation of leaders brought revitalized energy to the hospital's management, board, and professional staffs. Teaching and research activities increased, the hospital began to move closer to academia, and innovations were introduced in medicine, surgery, and patient care. Moreover, the Deaconess operated at capacity, finances were healthy, and the staff remained strong and grew more cohesive. A derailed merger between the Deaconess and the Lahey Clinic in the early 1970s, however, exposed old fault lines, while raising worrisome questions about the hospital's future.

NEW LEADERSHIP

In January 1953, just as the new Central Building was nearing completion, Warren Cook suffered a heart attack and went on medical leave. Don Lowry, who had arrived seven years earlier as Cook's assistant, became acting director. Cook had worked long (approximately sixteen years) and hard to bring the Central Building to fruition. Although he attended the formal dedication in June, his health subsequently forced him to step down. A grateful Executive Committee extended Cook a generous salary as a fund-raising consultant, while naming Lowry to succeed him as executive director, effective January 1, 1954. Lowry had turned forty the previous November and remained the Deaconess's chief executive until his retirement in 1975. Between them, Cook and Lowry directed the hospital for forty-six years, well over half its life span when Lowry retired.

Trained in the military, Lowry was a thorough-going, professional hospital administrator. Unlike his predecessor, he was not a minister; he was not even a Methodist. In fact, he was a warden of an Episcopal church in Westwood, Massachusetts, where he lived. While Lowry was still acting director, Stanley MacMullen, chairman of the Executive Committee, had suggested that Lowry's appointment to the directorship would be facilitated by switching to Methodism. But Lowry stuck to his beliefs and the Executive Committee put aside its reservations. Not long after, when John Wesley Lord, the Methodist bishop for New England who was president of the hospital corporation, returned from a trip to Africa, he discovered a flood of messages and phone calls that had arrived from around the country protesting Lowry's appointment. Lord good-naturedly kidded Lowry that many church members wondered why there were seventy-two Methodist hospitals in the United States and that only one did not have a Methodist at the helm. The Deaconess continued to have sectarian representation on its board, but Lowry's appointment signified the hospital's continuing evolution toward non-sectarianism.

Bishop Lord remained on the Executive Committee until 1960, when he resigned because of a transfer to Washington. Subsequently, James K. Mathews, his successor as bishop in New England, became a member of the Deaconess Board of Trustees, though not of the Executive Committee, another sign of the waning sectarian involvement. Similarly, although the bylaw requiring that a majority of corporators belong to the Methodist Episcopal Church remained on the books until a revision in 1975, the rule had long been ignored in practice. Certain Methodist influences remained in evidence, to be sure. Shortly after he became director, Lowry was forced to fire public relations consultants after they had innocently proposed that the Executive Committee and doctors have a cocktail party to become better acquainted with one another. This suggestion offended the teetotaling chairman, Stanley MacMullen.

Like Cook, Lowry was vigorous, well-organized, and a superb spokesman for the Deaconess. He developed warm friendships and excellent working relationships with staff members, and he enjoyed walking through the hospital and visiting various departments. Lowry was receptive to new ideas and was always willing to try out new services, technologies, and approaches to patient care, particularly when trusted professionals at the Deaconess advocated them. He was a builder and innovator at a propitious time — the economy was flourishing, demand for hospital services was growing, and medical science and technology were burgeoning.

And like his predecessor, Lowry reported to the trustees' Executive Committee, which numbered twelve and met monthly. The committee was composed largely of businessmen, but contained at least one lawyer who served as clerk, first Vincent P. Clarke and then James T. Mountz. The committee usually included two doctors *ex officio* from the Medical Administrative Board who were elected by the staff. Membership was stable and seasoned, with relatively little turnover.

Frank Capper, who had been the hospital's treasurer from 1934 through 1952, served with remarkable dedication as corporation president from 1956 through 1964 and then as chairman of the board until 1972. He was greatly admired and respected throughout the institution. His protégé, Laurens (Laurie) MacLure, who served under him at Boston Safe Deposit and Trust Company, became assistant treasurer in 1956. MacLure was soon asked to join the Executive Committee, where he stood out by virtue of his youth — he was only in his mid-thirties when most Executive Committee members were twenty-five, thirty, or even forty years his senior. MacLure became committee president in 1965 at the tender age of forty. The following year C. Vincent (Vince) Vappi, a contemporary of MacLure and a prominent general contractor, joined him on the Executive Committee.

In 1967, following a consultant's review of hospital organization, Lowry advanced to the newly created position of executive vice president to oversee long-range planning, development, medical staff liaison, and external communications. Dick Lee, who had been associate director, assumed the director's position and was, in effect, chief operating officer. Both Lowry and Lee were highly regarded by their peers. And like Cook before them, both served terms as president of the Massachusetts Hospital Association.

These were years when third-party payments — from private insurance companies, Blue Cross, or, after the passage of Medicare in 1965, the federal government — began to have a profound impact on hospitals. At the Deaconess, patient days covered by third-party payments rose from 53 percent in 1955 to 97 percent in 1970. The availability of third-party payments and the expansion of coverage and benefits allowed, indeed encouraged, the Deaconess and other hospitals to spend on more and better patient care, new technologies, specializations and subspecializations, and improved and expanded facilities.

Among the innovations introduced during this time was automated record keeping. Hospitals began to rely on modern data processing systems and then computers to deal more efficiently with the flood of paperwork that was beginning to engulf them as a result of

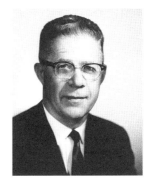

ROBERT D. LOWRY, CA. 1955. *For almost three decades, Lowry played an important role in the development of the modern Deaconess Hospital. Succeeding Warren Cook as executive director in 1954, Lowry guided the hospital through a period of physical expansion, staff consolidation, and scientific innovation.*

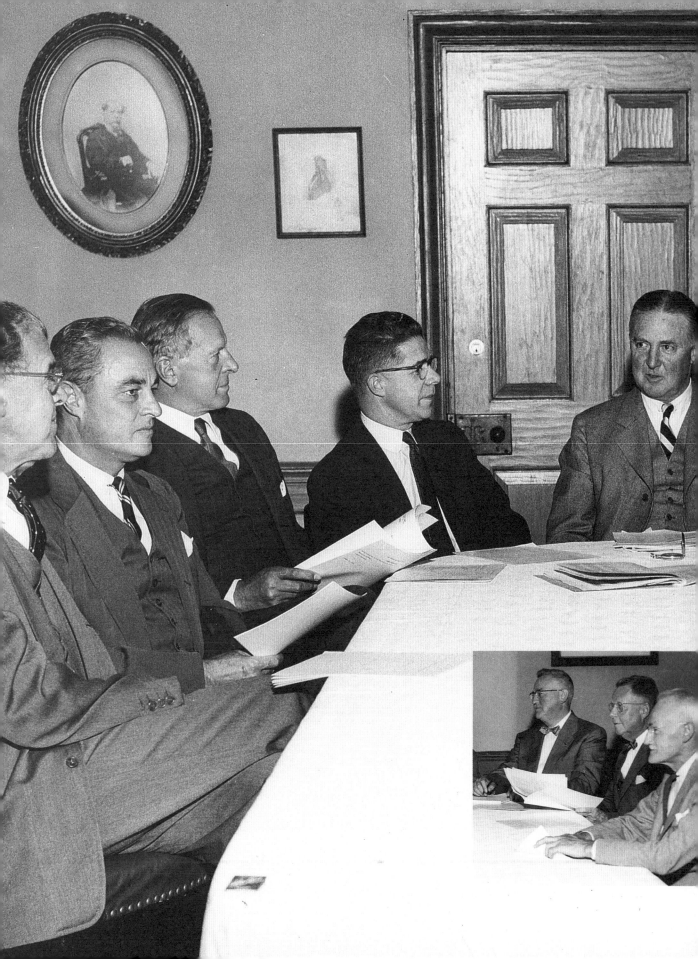

third-party payments. The Deaconess installed its first IBM equipment in 1960; in 1963 the hospital promoted itself as the first in the United States to install the IBM 1440, a "mechanical Colossus."

The growth of services was, of course, accompanied by an expansion of staff nationwide. "There were 150 full-time (equivalent) personnel for every 100 patients in 1946; up to 250 in 1965," historian Rosemary Stevens has noted. The number of employees at the Deaconess increased from 979 in 1960 to 1,331 in 1970. The hospital's operating expenses in 1953 were $2.7 million; twenty years later the figure had increased more than tenfold. Payroll constituted 56.9 percent of all expenses in 1950 and 62.2 percent in 1970. Because the Deaconess was a referral hospital, which cared for relatively ill patients, expense per bed ($46,755 in 1970) was high compared to the Massachusetts average ($32,532), but not far above the Boston average of $43,683. Massachusetts General's was the highest at $72,935. The expansion of staff and services, growing budgets, and increasingly complex relationships with payors led to commensurate growth in hospital administration. In 1953, the Deaconess had one assistant director, who, in fact, was the acting director; twenty years later, the administration included an executive vice president, a director, an associate director, and four assistant directors. Administrative costs of all kinds increased from 7.2 percent of total expenses in 1950 to 11.4 percent in 1970.

AFTER HE BECAME EXECUTIVE VICE PRESIDENT, Lowry continued to oversee the New England Deaconess School of Nursing, in which he always took a keen interest. This role kept him in touch with Ellen D. Howland, the director of nursing, with whom he had a close friendship and an excellent working relationship. Howland, a 1942 graduate of the school and a descendant of a New Bedford whaling captain, had been the school's assistant director in 1956 when Lowry asked her to become acting director of nursing until he could find a permanent replacement. She reluctantly agreed; Lowry later recalled that he never even looked for anybody else. He kept telling Howland that she would be perfect for the job. "Well, I am perfect," she would sardonically respond, "but not perfect for this job." She finally relented.

MEMBERS OF THE EXECUTIVE COMMITTEE, CA. 1954. *Executive Committee meetings were held in the Charles Dickens Room of the Parker House in downtown Boston.*

In large photograph, from left, Dr. Richard B. Cattell, Henry S. Rogerson, William B. Snow, Robert D. Lowry, and Francis W. Capper (chairman).

Inset, from left, Vincent P. Clarke, John Barnard, and Alfred E. Gardner.

Howland not only *was* perfect for the job, she was a perfectionist. A hard master on herself, she was forgiving of others' errors — at least up to a point. Gracious and proper, Howland also possessed a keen and, at moments, wicked sense of humor. She had literally hundreds of friends, a remarkable memory for people, names, and dates, and was active and highly respected in the nursing profession. She wanted every Deaconess graduate to be superior, not just adequate, was constantly striving for ways to improve the school, and was dedicated to the principle that nursing existed to help patients.

During Howland's early years as nursing director, she made it a point to visit patients who were in the hospital for more than a few days. She was devoted to "*The* New England Deaconess Hospital," as she usually referred to it; the initials, NEDH, by coincidence, also stood for Nurse Ellen D. Howland, as friends sometimes pointed out and teased her. She later remembered that the only time she ever had an argument with Lowry, he told her, "Now you're talking like a nurse." "Well, that's what I am," Howland matter-of-factly replied, and that was the end of the argument.

Moreover, Howland virtually personified the hospital and became a walking authority on its history and traditions. In 1967 she was made an assistant director of the Deaconess, thereby becoming part of the hospital's top management team a decade or more ahead of her counterparts in many hospitals and well before the American Hospital Association endorsed the idea of having directors of nursing included in upper-level management. Howland's inclusion was due to the Deaconess's particular history, to her own personal attributes and relationships with people, and to Lowry's appreciation of the importance of patient care.

From the hospital's founding, nursing and patient care had been central to its mission and, under Howland's leadership, they remained so. The nursing school continued to provide the Deaconess with a steady stream of highly skilled nurses. Its students routinely scored at or very near the top of the statewide exams that were administered upon graduation. Doctors and patients alike appreciated the excellent bedside skills of Deaconess-trained nurses. Although many graduates stayed on at the hospital as staff nurses (over one-third of the staff were alumni), some preferred to go elsewhere after their training or to seek additional education. The staffing needs grew to such an extent that the hospital had to hire more alumni of other schools. Despite the hospital's reputation for hiring its own, many non-Deaconess graduates became valued members of the staff and nursing administration.

By the 1960s the direction of nursing education began to shift away from diploma schools toward collegiate programs. Between 1956 and 1962, the number of baccalaureate nursing programs increased from 161 to 178, and average enrollment grew from 116 to 132. Correspondingly, diploma nursing schools declined from 1,134 in 1949 to 875 in 1964. Rather than save hospitals money, diploma schools were now a drain on finances. But Lowry as well as many key Deaconess doctors believed that the New England Deaconess School of Nursing helped define the hospital's essential character. A long-range study of the Deaconess nursing school in 1967 reaffirmed the hospital's commitment to its diploma school while proposing a number of specific measures to assure that its students, faculty, tuition, and education would remain competitive.

In 1963, the School of Nursing ended its fifty-year relationship with Simmons College and affiliated with Northeastern University, enabling students to receive college credit and work toward bachelor's degrees. Northeastern also provided more course offerings and more space for Deaconess students. In addition, it became quite common for graduates of the Deaconess nursing school to complete their bachelor's and master's degrees at Boston University.

In 1961, a task force appointed by the United States Surgeon General had recommended, among other things, an expansion of nursing schools within colleges and universities. The task force also encouraged growth in the number of nurses with master's or higher degrees. Because of these changes in accreditation, nursing students no longer provided an inexpensive source of labor.

In response, the federal government passed the Nurse Training Act of 1964 under which diploma, associate-degree, and baccalaureate and graduate schools of nursing were eligible to receive grants. The government also authorized long-term, low-interest student loans. The Deaconess, like most hospitals, relied primarily on staff nurses, but employed growing numbers of other trained workers as well — X-ray and laboratory technicians, physical and occupational therapists, social workers, dietitians, licensed practical nurses, nurses' aides, and

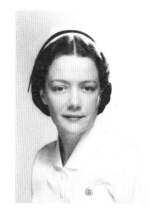

ELLEN D. HOWLAND, CA. 1956. *The granddaughter of a New Bedford whaling captain, Howland graduated from the New England Deaconess Hospital School of Nursing in 1942 and served the hospital as Director of Nursing Service and the School of Nursing from 1956 until her retirement in 1985.*

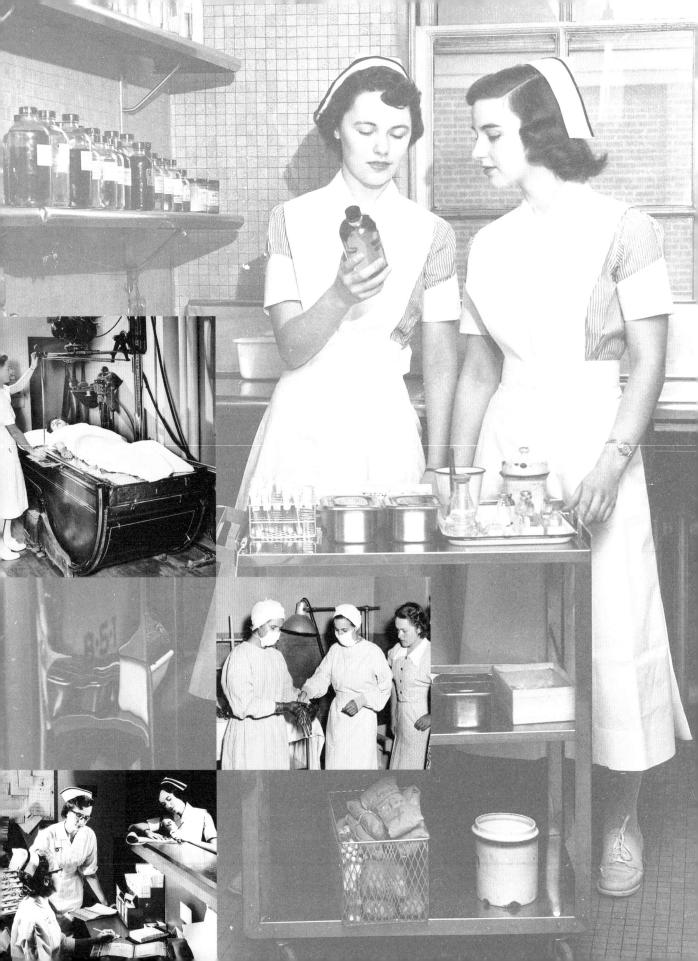

others. In 1950, the Deaconess had two employees per bed; in 1970, it had 3.77. In 1950, there were .54 nursing personnel per bed; in 1970, 1.30.

During these years, the booming health industry and shortages in certain kinds of trained personnel led to a high turnover rate and rising wages and benefits. The Deaconess managed to keep its turnover rate "down" to 33 percent or so in the early 1960s, for example, by offering competitive salaries, a good environment, and challenging work.

DURING THIS PERIOD SIGNIFICANT CHANGES were also taking place within the Deaconess medical staff. Despite suffering from advanced heart disease, knowledge of which he kept to himself, Frank Lahey continued to perform surgery into his seventies. In June 1953, while operating at New England Baptist Hospital, he suffered a severe heart attack. His death, which came within two weeks, accelerated a pre-existing crisis within the Lahey Clinic over succession. Apparently with the backing of Lahey, Linda Strand, the clinic's longtime business manager, had quietly arranged to take over as president and director herself, pushing aside Richard Cattell. Lahey had designated Cattell as his successor on a number of occasions, although, perhaps in part because of the deterioration in his own health, he had also shown animosity and jealousy toward the younger man.

Horrified by this unexpected turn of events, the Lahey Clinic medical staff mounted a challenge. By November 1953 they had convinced Lahey's widow, Alice, to vote to oust Strand. After Alice Lahey resigned as a clinic trustee herself, new trustees, predominantly doctors, were elected and chose Cattell as president. Strand would not give up so easily, however. When she refused to leave the clinic, Cattell actually had to have the sheriff evict her. It was soon discovered that many records were missing. More troubling, Strand produced a statement that had been signed by Lahey himself substantiating her claims to life-time employment and to certain remuneration. She sued, and in 1962 the clinic settled her claim.

Although this imbroglio was expensive for the clinic and caused great anxiety and consternation, it inflicted no other harm. Frank Lahey had attracted many outstanding specialists who developed fulfilling careers and they stayed with the clinic through this crisis. Moreover,

DEACONESS NURSES *in various phases of training during the late 1940s and early 1950s. From the beginning School of Nursing students were taught to uphold the highest standards of the nursing profession. Through the years Deaconess-trained nurses earned a reputation for providing highly skilled and compassionate care.*

Cattell, who served as director until 1962, accepted a degree of management participation by staff doctors that Lahey himself would probably have found intolerable. The democratization continued under Herbert Adams, who succeeded Cattell as director and served in this position until 1969.

The days of proprietary ownership of group practices or whole clinics were ending; the Lahey Clinic's outstanding doctors would have had no trouble finding fulfilling employment elsewhere or could have gone into practice for themselves if they ever became dissatisfied. Moreover, the clinic's continued growth through the 1950s and 1960s virtually required a broader sharing of authority since it would have been impossible for one person to do everything that Frank Lahey had once done. By 1964 the clinic's leading doctors, realizing that the legal structure had to be altered and that they needed top-level business assistance as well, hired Donald McLean as president. A lawyer by training, McLean had previously worked for the Rockefeller Foundation in New York, helped reorganize the Cleveland Clinic, and had been president of Overlook Hospital in Summit, New Jersey.

At the Joslin, succession proceeded much more smoothly. Elliott Joslin had been the sole proprietor of his practice, but in 1952 he formally organized the Joslin Clinic, naming Howard Root clinical director and Alexander Marble research director. Joslin's selflessness is illustrated by an experience veteran Joslin physician Leo Krall has recalled. In 1954, after Krall had been at the clinic as a young doctor for a year, Joslin offered him a magnificent raise of $1,500. Krall wondered where the money would come from. "At my age, I'm fortunate to be alive," replied Joslin. "You take $1,000 of mine and Dr. Howard Root will pay $500 of his."

Remarkably, Joslin continued to see patients until two days before he died peacefully in 1962 at the age of ninety-two. And he remained parsimonious to the end. Shortly before his death, Joslin observed the production of a movie on diabetes being filmed at the clinic. Huge lights illuminated the scene. Joslin could not understand what they were for; after their presence was explained, he asked in true New England Yankee fashion: "Well, can't you turn them off while we're talking? Who's paying for the electricity?"

Staff consolidation

During these years the Deaconess medical staff began to move, however slowly, toward consolidation. New staff bylaws, which had been drafted by Lyman Hoyt, took effect in 1951, reorganizing the Deaconess division and the Palmer division into the medical staff of New England Deaconess Hospital. These bylaws were revised several times in ensuing years. Under the 1951 revision a hospital administrative staff was created, chaired by Cattell and comprising Frank Allan (of the Lahey Clinic), Lyman Hoyt, Joseph Marks, Leland McKittrick, Howard Root, and Shields Warren. Hoyt was named physician-in-chief, while McKittrick became surgeon-in-chief. This board was subsequently expanded and included representatives from the general medical and general surgical divisions, the Joslin and Lahey clinics, and the Departments of Pathology and Radiology.

The hospital's new Medical Administrative Board (the official appellation) determined who was to be admitted to the staff. In practice both Lahey and Joslin doctors received privileges by virtue of their clinic affiliations, so the board actually only chose the independents. Because Joslin and Lahey staff members had first call on a majority of the hospital's beds, independent doctors were not eager to expand their own numbers for that would increase demand and competition. On occasion they did bring in assistants who went on the associate staff, however. In time, some of the associates moved up to the active or senior staff. Despite the modest step toward unification in 1951, however, the Lahey surgeons continued to control their own dedicated operating rooms until the mid-1960s.

While the Deaconess was taking its first steps toward consolidation of the medical staff, national accreditation committees and boards were requiring hospitals to amalgamate services and to appoint chairmen of medicine and surgery; so, too, would any medical school with which the Deaconess might wish to affiliate. But the Deaconess did not leap into filling these appointments with enthusiasm. The chairmanship in medicine was filled by the leading internal candidate only after he had accepted a prestigious position outside Boston, while the surgery position was assumed by an internal candidate from the Lahey Clinic, despite the qualms of independent surgeons.

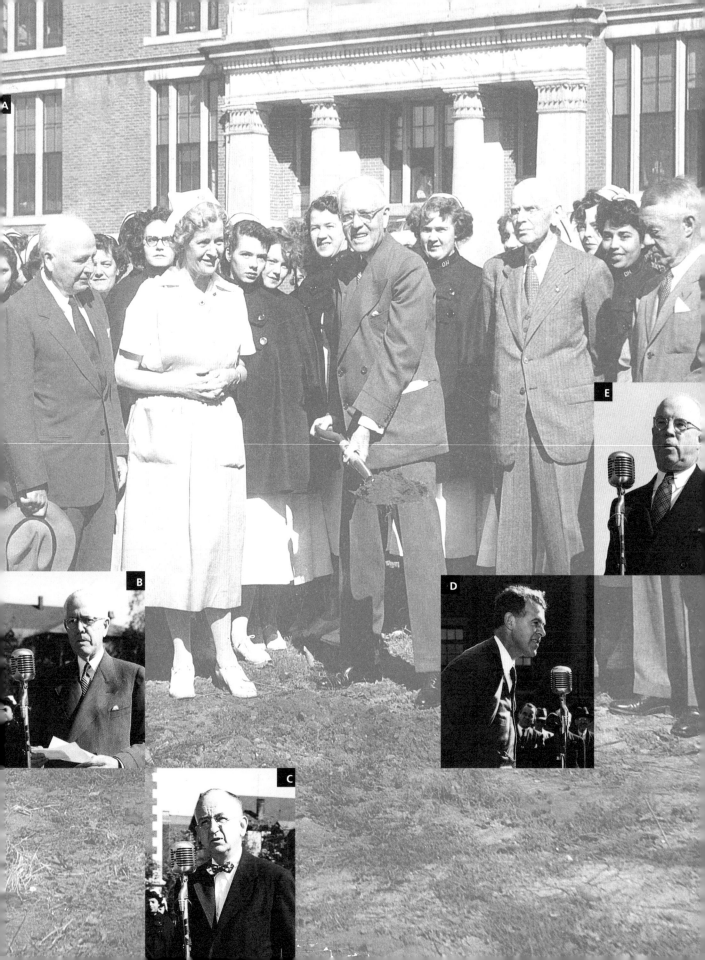

The new chairman of medicine, James L. Tullis, had spent several years as an assistant to Gorham Brigham. After leaving Brigham's practice, he began to conduct important research in hematology, became an assistant professor of medicine at Harvard, and spent considerable time teaching at Peter Bent Brigham Hospital. Tullis was highly regarded by Hoyt, by Robert Bradley, who succeeded Howard Root as the Joslin's medical director, and by other leading internists at the Deaconess, where he was also a member of the active staff. In fact, Tullis chaired the general medical division of the Medical Administrative Board in the early 1960s. In 1964, after Tullis was offered and accepted a job as chief of medicine at Roosevelt Hospital in New York and as professor of medicine at Columbia University, the Deaconess responded by asking him to chair a new Department of Medicine. Tullis accepted, largely because his family had resisted moving to New York. He brought his Harvard-supported laboratory to the hospital and divided his time between research, practicing medicine, and overseeing the nascent department, about which a number of independent staff members were, from the start, skeptical and suspicious.

Following Tullis's appointment, Leland McKittrick became interim chairman of surgery while a search began for a permanent leader. It was McKittrick who took the first important steps toward staff unification. "For the first time in the history of the Hospital," he reported in 1965, "the entire Surgical Staff has met monthly, and the meetings have been well received. The recently established weekly conferences of the surgical residents and members of the Surgical Staff, during which all complications in patients on the General Surgical Service are critically reviewed, have proven stimulating and instructive." McKittrick, of course, like outstanding Deaconess independents from Massachusetts General and other teaching hospitals, had liked the fact that the Deaconess was not a teaching hospital. But he also recognized that times were changing and that the Deaconess would have to change too.

The search committee did not have to look far to find the ideal candidate for the surgery post. One of the Lahey Clinic's finest and busiest surgeons, Cornelius E. (Neil) Sedgwick, was also an excellent teacher. Coincidentally, Sedgwick was an old friend of Jim Tullis. Both had started as interns on the same day at Roosevelt Hospital in New

A GROUND-BREAKING CEREMONIES *for the new Central Building, October 20, 1950. Participating in the festivities were represen- tatives of the Deaconess board, employees, administration, volunteers, and nursing and medical staff, including*

B ERNEST G. HOWES, *President of the Corporation*

C STANLEY O. MACMULLEN, *Chairman, Executive Committee*

D DR. RICHARD B. CATTELL, *Surgeon-in-Chief*

E DR. HOWARD F. ROOT, *Physician-in-Chief*

York and had then been drafted into military service at the same time and even served part of the war together. By pure happenstance they had both ended up in Boston and on the Deaconess staff. The fact that Tullis and Sedgwick liked each other and were old friends facilitated good working relations.

Initially, independent surgeons expressed anxiety about the selection of a Lahey staff member as surgeon-in-chief: would he give preference to the Lahey Clinic in assigning operating room time? At one meeting, George W. B. Starkey, an independent thoracic surgeon, assured wary independents that they would never have anything to worry about with Sedgwick, whom he knew well. When McKittrick and Roger Graves interviewed the future chairman, they asked about the potential of divided loyalty. Sedgwick turned the tables and replied that he would only accept the job if he had their full personal support. The offer was made and McKittrick and Graves backed Sedgwick steadfastly from that time on.

Sedgwick, in fact, never demonstrated the slightest favoritism toward the Lahey Clinic and, if anything, bent over backward in favor of the independents. He was, in the view of vascular surgeon Frank Wheelock, "wonderful," and Wheelock's view typified the attitude of the entire surgical staff. The Deaconess paid the Lahey Clinic for Sedgwick's services, though he never knew how much, at least not until later when Laurie MacLure told him the hospital wanted to give him a raise and wanted to be sure that he actually received it.

Building upon the foundation that McKittrick had laid, Sedgwick, who officially became chairman on February 1, 1966, consolidated the surgical department further. He ended the old practice of having separate operating rooms for the Lahey Clinic and expanded ties which had been established in the early 1960s with Harvard's Fifth Surgical Service at Boston City Hospital. Sedgwick also reorganized the cardiovascular thoracic service, combining the specialists in that area from the Lahey, Overholt Clinic, and the general staff. In addition, he helped develop a tumor conference and clinic and held weekly meetings of the surgical staff.

Perhaps because of Sedgwick's Lahey affiliation, it was a little easier to achieve cohesion and consolidation in surgery than it was in medicine. Since the Joslin Clinic had chosen not to hire surgeons, there were only two groups of surgeons to bring together — Lahey and the independents. Joslin physicians referred surgical cases, many of them involving foot and vascular problems, to Deaconess independents including Clifford Franseen, Carl Hoar, Leland McKittrick, John McKittrick (Leland's brother), Theodore Pratt, and Frank Wheelock.

In medicine, on the other hand, there were three separate groups, Lahey, Joslin, and the general staff. Since Tullis was himself one of the independents, a quite diffuse group, he functioned from a more difficult position than Sedgwick. Nevertheless, Tullis did manage to build an accredited residency program in the 1960s and initiated an exchange of residents with Peter Bent Brigham Hospital. Important allies in the latter effort were George Thorn and later Eugene Braunwald, chiefs of medicine at the Brigham and full-time professors of medicine at Harvard. Under the Harvard system, it was they, not Tullis, who had the authority to make clinical teaching appointments at the Deaconess.

Changes in the Department of Pathology were achieved more easily. In 1963 leadership in pathology was assumed by William Meissner when Shields Warren formally stepped down. (Warren remained with the hospital as head of a cancer research organization until 1968 and was succeeded in 1969 by George Nichols, who served but a few years.) Meissner had for some time essentially run the pathology department, including its well-known residency program, in consultation with Warren, whom he greatly admired. Like Warren, Meissner was a respected scientist, a professor at Harvard, and extremely loyal to the Deaconess — both Warren and Meissner periodically wrote checks to the hospital drawn from the department's surpluses. Bright, congenial, good-humored, and a thorough gentleman, Meissner was a beloved figure at the Deaconess.

The surpluses generated in pathology came from the clinical pathology lab, which became ever busier — automated equipment was enhancing laboratory productivity significantly. In addition to providing services to the Deaconess, the clinical lab also continued to be utilized by New England Baptist and other hospitals.

The clinical lab was run during these years by Bradley E. Copeland, who became an international leader in quality control. In 1961, in cooperation with Northeastern University, Copeland created a School of Medical Technology at the Deaconess for training college-educated laboratory technicians, apparently the first such program in the

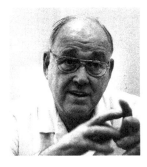

DR. CORNELIUS E. (NEIL) SEDGWICK, 1977. *A superbly gifted surgeon on the Lahey Clinic staff, Sedgwick succeeded McKittrick as chief of Deaconess surgery in 1966. Following McKittrick's lead, Sedgwick further consolidated the Department of Surgery, ending the practice of separate facilities for the Lahey and general surgical staffs.*

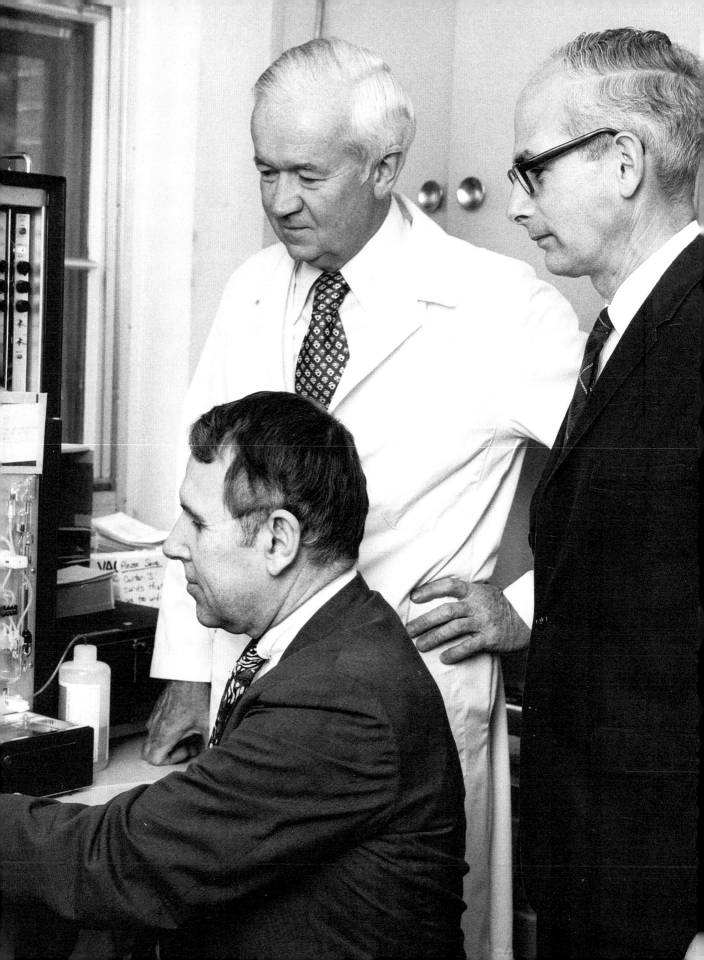

United States. Some of the school's alumni staffed the hospital's own clinical laboratory, one of Copeland's central purposes in starting the school. Copeland held an academic appointment at Northeastern, as did Meissner.

IN THE EARLY 1960S, Lowry and the hospital's top independent doctors, particularly Hoyt and Graves, decided to expand and upgrade the hospital's small residency programs, which had been initiated in 1957. They believed that if the hospital were to stay in the forefront of medical science and patient care and if it were to continue to attract an outstanding staff, vibrant residency programs would be essential, especially in Boston, a center of medical education. "We have had internationally known men on our staff in the past, and we have many at the present time," Lowry wrote in the 1961 Deaconess report. "But what about the future?"

Hospital residents were given significant responsibility for special twenty-six-bed teaching units in medicine and surgery in Palmer, subsequently named for Hoyt and Graves. Patients in these areas typically were unable to afford a professional fee. Since the Deaconess lacked an emergency room from which these units might draw patients, they were dependent upon staff doctors for referrals. The sections were augmented by the Richard Thaler Unit on another Palmer floor, dedicated to the memory of a young Deaconess physician who had been active in the organization of a teaching service.

Most staff doctors were reluctant to turn over responsibility for fee-paying patients to residents, though some were amenable. However, these same physicians generally welcomed having residents around to deal with patient emergencies when they themselves were unavailable. By 1970, in addition to training pathology residents, the Deaconess had a residency program in internal medicine, with fellowship programs in subspecialties in diabetic care, cardiology, and hematology. There were also a small number of residents in thoracic surgery, urology, and therapeutic radiology. Overall, the house staff expanded from fifteen to fifty between 1960 and 1971. In 1970 residency programs cost the Deaconess more than $500,000.

DEACONESS PATHOLOGY LEADERSHIP, 1972. Standing from left, Dr. William A. Meissner, Dr. Merle A. Legg, and Dr. Bradley E. Copeland (seated). Following Meissner's retirement as department chairman in 1972 (he remained as pathologist and Harvard professor), the position rotated between Copeland and Legg. Upon Copeland's departure in 1979, Legg assumed all duties as chairman of the Deaconess Department of Pathology and continued until his own retirement from full-time responsibilities in 1989.

A TRIAL MARRIAGE

In 1968 Tullis chaired a Deaconess committee to explore medical school affiliation for the hospital. Lowry, MacLure, Meissner, Sedgwick, and two other members of the Executive Committee, Albert Pratt and James F. Farr, also served. They met with senior members of the staff and with representatives of various medical schools in New England and elsewhere. Although many area institutions were interested in forming an alliance with the Deaconess, the staff favored a Harvard affiliation. A number of staff members held Harvard teaching appointments and participated in the instruction of medical students. The hospital's pathology department was already a full-scale affiliate of Harvard as was the Division of Therapeutic Radiology. Of course, Harvard was also widely regarded as among the best medical schools in the country, if not the world, and was the alma mater of quite a few staff physicians.

While preferring a Harvard affiliation, the general staff wanted a loose association that would preserve the Deaconess's independence as well as their own. Staff doctors certainly were not interested in accepting Harvard's regulation of their incomes; nor were they prepared to give up firm control of patient care. Some worried privately about whether they would pass muster at Harvard for clinical appointments.

Robert H. Ebert, dean of Harvard Medical School, was willing to accept a loose arrangement since Harvard, unique in this respect, was accustomed to having flexible relationships with its hospitals. Harvard had no formal written contracts with any of its affiliated institutions and the hospitals were free to accept as much or as little regulation from Harvard as they wanted. The medical school did firmly control academic appointments, however. A hospital could name a new chief of surgery, for example, without the approval of Harvard's medical faculty and its dean, but Harvard could then deny the person a professorship and could strip the hospital of a Harvard-endowed chair, if it had one.

Ebert was also prepared to proceed with the Deaconess on a department-by-department basis. Thus, by early 1970, the Deaconess, both trustees and staff, agreed to a "trial marriage" without a binding commitment by either party. The short prenuptial agreement that accompanied the affiliation made clear that neither side was making a major commitment — no obligations were spelled out and any alliances that developed were subject to approval by both institutions. The agreement was obviously intended to allay suspicions by the medical staff that Harvard was taking over either the Deaconess or them.

BUILDING EXPANSION AND PROGRAM INNOVATION

The hospital campus changed and grew significantly between the early 1950s and early 1970s, as aerial photographs of the Longwood medical area vividly illustrate. Expansion was spurred by demand, but it was made possible by the availability of funding, which came primarily through loans, contributions, and federal grants. Growth also reflected vision and the willingness of the administration to try new things and to take risks. It was here that the hospital's leadership chose to forge ahead rather than march in place. Expansion was not entirely accomplished by New England Deaconess Hospital alone, but also by institutions closely related and proximate to it. Appropriately enough, hospital publications began to refer to the "New England Deaconess Complex."

In 1951, the Cancer Research Institute (CRI) was built with nearly $500,000 in federal funds that Shields Warren had secured. At its opening, the institute included an outpatient cancer clinic of Deaconess Hospital, the Cancer Control Division of the Harvard School of Public Health, the Tumor Diagnosis Service of the Harvard Cancer Commission, and experimental research laboratory groups in biochemistry, biophysics, radiobiology, hematology, and pathology. Over the next twenty years, CRI was supported entirely by government contracts and grants and by foundation awards. Its work focused primarily on research and spawned hundreds of scientific papers. CRI attracted a number of distinguished scientists in addition to Warren, including W. Eugene Knox, a professor of biological chemistry at Harvard Medical School.

Housed in the Cancer Research Institute was a 250-seat auditorium named for Elliott Joslin. Doctors personally raised most of the money toward building and furnishing this facility, contributing generously because of their great admiration and respect for Joslin. The auditorium was subsequently used for teaching diabetic patients and for a variety of other instructional purposes, including grand rounds.

The auditorium proved a valuable addition, particularly as the hospital evolved into a teaching institution. Another asset, the Gilbert Horrax Memorial Library, which opened in 1959 on the first floor of the Deaconess Building, was named in honor of the hospital's first staff neurosurgeon.

The completion of the Central Building in 1953 increased beds at the hospital to 375 and centralized a number of services. Financing for the structure was derived from three sources: $1.5 million in contributions, $1.5 million in a mortgage from John Hancock, and a $410,000 grant from the federal government. The contributions were raised through voluntary quotas on three groups — the corporation and trustees; doctors, whose percentages were based on fee-for-service over the previous five years; and the Methodist Church, whose New England congregations contributed nominal sums. The federal grant was awarded under the Hill-Burton Act of 1946, a landmark piece of legislation in American hospital history. Under Hill-Burton, the federal government helped finance construction at thousands of hospitals, though almost half of the grants were directed to communities with populations under 10,000. Attached to the Central Building was a non-denominational chapel made possible through a $100,000 donation secured by Don Lowry from Arthur T. Dooley. Dooley himself was a Christian Scientist and as such would not support a hospital building per se. Dooley donated the chapel as a memorial to his late wife, an even more ardent Christian Scientist.

In 1953, the year that the Central Building opened, the Deaconess also established an electroshock therapy ward on the first floor of the Deaconess Building. Controversial ever since its arrival in the United States from Hungary in the 1930s, electroshock therapy was generally frowned upon by psychoanalysts, who were then in the ascendancy in psychiatry, and by many other doctors as well because the modality carried a significant mortality rate at the time. Consequently, its use was not accepted in many general facilities and tended to be restricted to psychiatric hospitals. In Boston, the two exceptions were the Deaconess and St. Elizabeth's Hospital.

At the Deaconess, Tillman McDaniel and Lyman Hoyt in particular recognized the value of electroshock therapy for some of their patients and were instrumental in recruiting Robert Fleming, a well-known Harvard-affiliated psychiatrist, to join the staff. A specialist in the treatment of alcoholism, Fleming was a pioneer in Boston in the use of electroshock treatment for patients with depression. Other psychiatrists soon joined Fleming in providing this treatment, including independents Oscar Raeder and Jackson Thomas, and Walter Tucker, head of psychiatry at the Lahey Clinic, who had pioneered in the use of lobotomies, a radical surgical procedure that later fell into disrepute.

Recognizing the value of electroshock therapy, Lowry took the lead in seeing to the acquisition in 1958 of the Channing Home, a recently closed, private, twenty-eight-bed tuberculosis sanatorium for women, adjacent to the hospital on Pilgrim Road. Because the purchase by the Deaconess had been made possible by the estate of Samuel Norwich, the new facility was renamed in his honor. Following renovations, the first floor was opened as an electroshock therapy unit in early 1959. The second level accommodated nineteen inpatients who, because they were ambulatory, were charged a lower daily rate than patients in the main hospital. Electroshock therapy was in such demand, however, that Norwich House could not accommodate all of the hospital's psychiatric patients, a number of whom continued to be housed across the street in the Central Building. Fleming reportedly led the Deaconess staff in admittances for a number of years.

IN THE MID-1950s, two more additions to the Deaconess complex were completed which were not actually part of the hospital itself. In 1955, Richard Overholt moved the Overholt Thoracic Clinic, a private practice on Beacon Street, to Francis Street and a new two-story office building designed in the International Style by Bauhaus architect Walter Gropius. Overholt's associates in these early years were Wilford B. Neptune, Norman J. Wilson, and Francis Woods. Overholt also sponsored a small residency program and hired its first graduate, James A. Bougas, who in 1956 assumed the leadership of a cardiac catheterization laboratory that Neptune had established at the Deaconess.

After moving to their new offices, the Overholt surgeons continued to perform surgery in tuberculosis sanatoria around New England, but new medications had begun to reduce dramatically the need for such procedures. Almost simultaneously, however, cardiac surgery came into its own. Both the Overholt Clinic and the Deaconess had several talented and skilled cardiothoracic specialists. Neptune, who had trained in Philadelphia under Charles Bailey, a pioneer in cardiothoracic

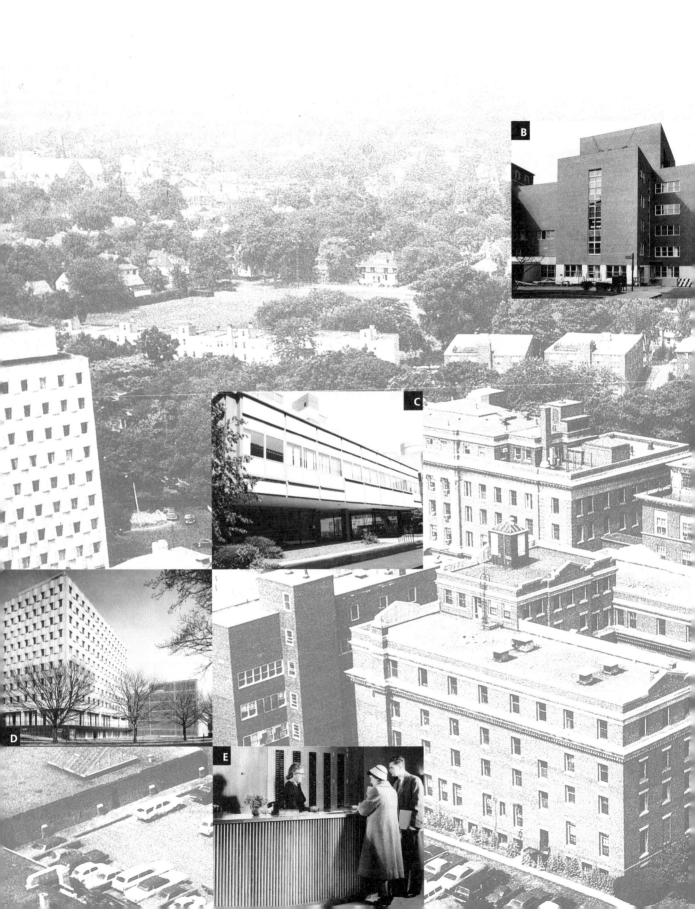

surgery, started performing open-heart surgery at the hospital in 1957 and made significant contributions to the development of the cardiopulmonary bypass and the use of the heart-lung machine and hemodilution. The Deaconess was among the first hospitals in Boston to perform this procedure. Also on the hospital staff were two cardiothoracic surgeons who were not affiliated with the Overholt Clinic. John W. Strieder had founded the thoracic surgery unit at Boston City Hospital in 1947, the first of its kind in New England. He was a professor at Boston University and became chairman of the American Board of Thoracic Surgery. George Starkey, a rising star, had received advanced training in London and at Children's Hospital in Boston.

In 1957 the Joslin Clinic relocated from Joslin's home at 81 Bay State Road to a new four-story structure diagonally across the street from the Deaconess Building on Pilgrim and Joslin Roads. Lowry had pleaded with Joslin to build foundations that would be strong enough to support additional floors, but Joslin did not have the money in hand and wanted, understandably enough, to live to see the building completed. Later, in the early 1960s, when funds became available, the two unfurnished top floors of the building were completed and equipped as laboratories for experimental work in diabetes. Dedicated as the Elliott P. Joslin Research Laboratory in 1964, the new facility on these floors became the successor to the Baker Clinical Laboratory at the Deaconess. Directed successively by Albert E. Renold and George F. Cahill, Jr., both full-time professors at Harvard Medical School, the Joslin lab conducted seminal research in metabolism and constituted another important link between the Deaconess and Harvard in these years.

While the new Joslin Clinic building was being planned, Lyman Hoyt had proposed to Joslin that he extend his building even higher to provide rental offices for physicians. The hospital's independent staff was spread all over the city and was spending increasing amounts of time traveling from place to place in Boston's steadily worsening traffic. Having the independent staff housed near the Deaconess, it was argued, would solidify their ties to the hospital and encourage concentration of their practices. Joslin was unpersuaded, however.

Around this time, Don Lowry also became an avid proponent of constructing a medical office building for the hospital's independent

A A VIEW OF DEACONESS HOSPITAL *from Brookline Avenue.*

B THE CENTRAL BUILDING, *completed in 1953.*

C OVERHOLT BUILDING, *a two-story office and ambulatory care building designed by renowned Bauhaus architect Walter Gropius.*

D LOWRY MEDICAL OFFICE BUILDING, *one of the first in the country to provide private office space for the independent members of a hospital staff. In the early years the building also housed motel rooms for families of out-of-town hospital patients.*

E LOBBY INFORMATION DESK *in the new Central Building, 1953.*

staff and it was he who brought the idea to fruition. Lowry believed that it would forge the independents' loyalty to the Deaconess. Independent staff members *were* independent; they had staff affiliations elsewhere and many sent patients, even a majority of their patients, to other hospitals. Lowry inspected medical office buildings in other cities, but there were none in Boston to match what he had in mind — a building dedicated to the practices of independent physicians.

In 1959, a parcel of land situated on Francis Street, Brookline Avenue, and the Riverway suddenly came up for sale. Lorande (Lorrie) M. Woodruff, a hospital urologist, wrote a personal check to keep the Deaconess in the bidding for the property until Lowry could get authorization to proceed. The parcel had been owned by the Donnelly advertising family in a revocable trust and the land itself had long been the site of one of many billboards along the Riverway. The billboard generated considerable revenues for the land's owners, but obscured the Deaconess and was considered an eyesore. Lowry encountered some skepticism among the trustees about investing hospital funds in a private office building, particularly one that might benefit doctors. But Lowry persevered and the Deaconess outbid a competitor and purchased the land for $175,000.

The building itself was financed in part by endowment funds and more than double that proportion by a mortgage on the land. Built at a cost of $4.3 million and completed in 1964, the 10-story office building and 300-space parking garage proved great assets. All available offices were quickly rented to physicians, most from the Deaconess staff, and a waiting list had to be established. The building included motel rooms for families of patients, operated at low cost by the hospital: half the Deaconess's patients came from outside the Boston area. The parking garage was also very busy and very profitable. Not only did the new building turn into a lucrative investment for the Deaconess, it also fulfilled Lowry's original purpose — enabling independent staff physicians to concentrate their practices in one convenient location, thereby strengthening their ties to the hospital.

CHANGE CONTINUED TO ALTER the face and direction of Deaconess Hospital over the next decade. In the early 1960s, Shields Warren was instrumental in raising $2.5 million in government and private grants for a radiation research laboratory. Completed in 1965, the new facility, appropriately enough, was named for its guiding force, Warren himself. The location of the Shields

Warren Radiation Laboratory on the corner of Brookline Avenue and
Binney Street put it at some remove from the rest of the hospital. In fact,
it was not exclusively a Deaconess undertaking. Although built and owned
by the Deaconess, the laboratory was actually a joint endeavor with Beth
Israel Hospital, Children's Hospital, and Harvard Medical School. Serving
as the first director was Professor Henry I. Kohn of Harvard Medical
School. Tunnels were excavated that eventually connected the Warren
laboratory to the Deaconess, to the other hospitals, except for Beth Israel,
and to the medical school. Links with the Harvard/Longwood medical
area were thus beginning to be put into place, not just programmatically,
but physically as well.

The collaborative nature of the Shields Warren laboratory
foreshadowed the later establishment of the Joint Center for Radiation
Therapy in 1968, for which Don Lowry, Joseph Marks, and Shields
Warren at the Deaconess, and Mitchell Rabkin at Beth Israel Hospital,
had helped lay the groundwork over a number of years. Through
Warren and Lowry nearly a decade earlier, the Deaconess had begun
to negotiate with the medical school for the appointment of a professor
of therapeutic radiology. Three years later the hospital agreed to participate in a salary guarantee for a full-time professor of radiation therapy
at Harvard. The Warren laboratory provided the Joint Center a base
of operations, though the endeavor was eventually a collaboration of four
hospitals, Beth Israel, Boston Hospital for Women, Peter Bent Brigham,
and the Deaconess, with Children's joining in 1971.

Samuel Hellman, who had been recruited from Yale by
Warren, Tullis, and Ebert, among others, and became professor of radiotherapy at Harvard, served very effectively as the Joint Center's first
chairman. Radiation therapy as well as chemotherapy were beginning
to demonstrate encouraging results against certain kinds of cancer.
In addition, radiation therapy involved very expensive equipment, so
pooling facilities and expertise made excellent sense economically,
as well as in terms of teaching and research, both important aspects of
the Joint Center's mission.

BY 1960 THE CENTRAL BUILDING WAS ALREADY beginning to prove inadequate for the hospital's needs, a recurring theme in the hospital's history.
Like many other institutions, the Deaconess had a higher proportion of

beds filled by medical patients than previously. In 1947, about 75 percent of the hospital's beds were taken up by surgical patients and 25 percent by medical cases. By 1962, the proportion was 40 percent surgical and 60 percent medical. The Deaconess consistently operated at more than 90 percent capacity throughout these years and had waiting lists; the national average for acute-care hospitals was 80 percent. The Lahey Clinic, which was growing steadily, clamored for more beds, but so did the general staff and the Joslin Clinic. In 1965 the Deaconess had 368 beds, including 189 in wards. That same year the hospital hired Dr. Anthony J. J. Rourke of New York, a leading hospital consultant, as an advisor. As is often the case, the consultant corroborated what the hospital's management already knew — that the Deaconess should expand once more. In consultation with Shepley Bulfinch Richardson and Abbott, the architectural firm that had designed the Central Building, and Turner Construction Company, which had built it, a plan was developed to add six floors to the Central Building, with a net increase of 129 beds, bringing the hospital's total to 497. The wing of the Central Building facing the Deaconess Building would be widened and extended to connect to the older structure.

In keeping with national trends, the building scheme proposed that the number of ward beds be reduced and semi-private rooms, which were now routinely paid for by insurers, increased, so that when construction was completed, there would be 113 private accommodations, 272 semi-private, and 112 ward. By 1967, 90 percent of Deaconess patients were covered by insurance. According to the original plan, the 139 beds in the Deaconess Building were to be discontinued in order to house service, teaching, and mechanical facilities. Designs called for the Deaconess Building to be razed without disrupting patient care when further expansion was necessary. As it turned out, however, clinical needs prevented the hospital from retiring the Deaconess Building from patient service.

THE PROPOSED HOSPITAL ADDITION must be seen in a larger context. This was a time of growing federal attention to hospitals and health care. President Lyndon B. Johnson, in his health and education message to Congress in March 1965, declared that one-third of the nation's hospital beds were in "obsolete condition." Medicare, health insurance for people over age sixty-five, financed through Social Security, was enacted in 1965, over the opposition of the American Medical Association and following a long struggle.

It was anticipated that Medicare would place significant additional demands on the nation's hospitals — and it did. "Medicare gave hospitals a license to spend," it has been observed, and spend they did. Of course, as government spending increased, so did regulation, a phenomenon that occurred irrespective of political party. Indeed, it was Republican President Richard M. Nixon who in 1971 imposed wage and price controls, including limits on hospitals, and at whose initiative legislation was enacted in 1973 to encourage the formation of health maintenance organizations.

The Massachusetts Health and Educational Facilities Authority, established in the late 1960s, allowed hospitals to obtain lower-cost financing through the issuance of tax-exempt bonds. That proved an important instrument for the Deaconess and for many other Massachusetts institutions. As with the federal government, growing state assistance was also accompanied in these years by increasing state regulation. By 1969 third-party reimbursements were being closely regulated by the Massachusetts Rate Setting Commission and, by 1973, new hospital facilities had to be approved by the Public Health Council of Massachusetts.

The estimated cost of the Central Building addition in 1965 was $8,150,000. Of this amount, $2.5 million was already in hand, a bequest from the estate of Frederick J. and Frank E. Farr. (This amount subsequently grew to $3.5 million.) Although patients of Tillman McDaniel in their old age, the Farr brothers, Brookline chemists, had never been Deaconess benefactors before; nor were they related to James F. Farr, a longtime trustee and member of the hospital's Executive Committee. One of the brothers' wives, however, had worked in Elliott Joslin's lab when she was young and had convinced them years before to put the Deaconess in their wills; after their deaths, she received an annuity from the hospital. In recognition of this munificent gift, in 1972 the Central Building was renamed the Farr Memorial Building.

The building program, which eventually included new operating suites and intensive care units (ICUs), also received funding from a number of other sources. The federal government provided

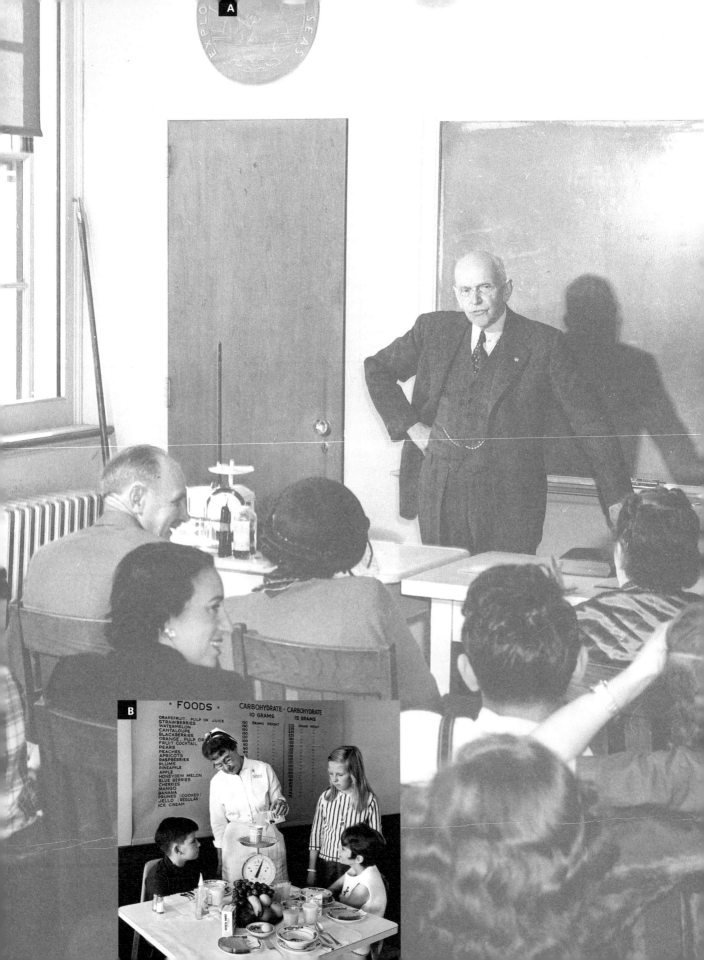

· FOODS ·   CARBOHYDRATE · CARBOHYDRATE
                            10 GRAMS   15 GRAMS

GRAPEFRUIT, PULP OR JUICE
STRAWBERRIES
WATERMELON
CANTALOUPE
BLACKBERRIES
ORANGE, PULP OR
FRUIT COCKTAIL
PEARS
PEACHES
APRICOTS
RASPBERRIES
PLUMS
PINEAPPLE
APPLE
HONEYDEW MELON
BLUE BERRIES
CHERRIES
MANGO
BANANA
PRUNES (COOKED)
JELLO (REGULAR)
ICE CREAM

$400,000 through a Hill-Burton grant. Several million dollars was raised in a capital campaign, including impressive contributions from independent and Overholt staff members ($343,000) and employees ($237,000), and institutional contributions from the Lahey and Joslin clinics ($500,000 and $250,000, respectively). Loans provided over a third of the needed funds. Borrowing for capital purposes was nothing new for the Deaconess, but long-term borrowing had now become commonplace among hospitals.

The Deaconess rebuilding program took longer than expected; it was logistically complex because all the work had to be accomplished in and around a busy hospital. A strike by ironworkers further delayed construction. By mid-summer 1971, however, all six of the new floors were in service. In 1972, other renovations were completed as was a new 415-car parking garage on the corner of Longwood Avenue and Autumn Street, at an additional cost of $2.5 million. The garage helped relieve what had become a chronic shortage of parking in the area.

By 1973 the Deaconess had two other capital projects in the works. A construction contract was let for a new clinical pathology laboratory and radiation therapy facility to be built on the site of Norwich House. Following a study reaffirming the hospital's commitment to the School of Nursing, the hospital had also begun to raise money for a new building to replace the antiquated Harris Hall. Both of these projects would come to fruition; neither of them included new patient beds.

With the completion of the new floors in the Farr Building in 1971, the hospital had close to 500 beds, employed 2,000 people, and had become one of the three or four largest hospitals in Boston. Celebrating its seventy-fifth anniversary that year, the hospital administration understandably took pride in how far the Deaconess had come from the fourteen-bed infirmary in the Massachusetts Avenue brownstone.

Yet despite its size and number of patients, the Deaconess was not that well known to many Bostonians since it was a specialty and referral hospital and drew patients from a wide geographic area. Two anecdotes illustrate the point. In 1953, when Warren Cook suffered a heart attack at home, Bob Brownlee called a police ambulance and instructed the officers to take Cook to the Deaconess. Brownlee even asked whether he should proceed first to show the way, but the police

A DR. ELLIOTT P. JOSLIN *conducting a patient education class in the basement of the Baker Clinic, ca. 1950. Joslin's commitment to educating patients never waned and earned him the title of "master clinician" of diabetes.*

B A NURSE TRAINED IN DIABETIC PATIENT EDUCATION *instructs young patients in proper dietary regimen in the new Hospital Teaching Unit, located in the Joslin Clinic and run by members of the Deaconess staff.*

assured him that they knew where it was. When Brownlee himself arrived at the hospital a little later, there was no evidence of either the ambulance or Cook. After a while he went outside as the ambulance came screeching up to the entrance. It turned out that the police had taken Cook to the Peter Bent Brigham; he had even been put to bed before the error was discovered.

Nineteen years later, prior to taking a teaching position at the School of Nursing, Judith R. Miller, who later became the hospital's chief nurse, has recalled driving by the Deaconess on a daily basis for a full year without ever being aware of its existence. The Deaconess, it was sometimes said, was the "best-kept secret in town."

Advances in patient care

Innovation in patient care has long played an important part in medicine. Throughout its history, the Deaconess has borrowed and adapted new methods and approaches from other institutions while breaking new ground of its own. Since ideas spread rapidly through medicine and people are constantly improving upon and refining the innovations of others, "firsts" can be hard to prove definitively. If not first, the Deaconess was certainly in the forefront in many areas of patient care and medical and surgical procedures in the decades following World War II.

In 1956, largely at the initiative of the nursing department, the Deaconess opened a thirteen-bed special care unit in a converted ward in the Deaconess Building. An early intensive care unit, the name "special care" was chosen, according to Ellen Howland, because it sounded a little more like nursing and a little less medical. Patients were considered for admission if their condition required frequent or unusual treatment, extensive or complicated nursing care and/or constant observation. A year after the unit opened, Leland McKittrick was able to tell the surgical staff that the new facility was saving an average of one life a week. To conform to national standards, the special care unit was later renamed an intensive care unit.

In 1957, the Deaconess opened the Hospital Teaching Unit for ambulatory diabetic patients. Located on the second floor of the Joslin Clinic, the facility was the fulfillment of a dream for Elliott Joslin. By prearrangement, the Deaconess administered the unit, which originally had forty beds and later increased to seventy; since patients were ambulatory and able to accomplish much for themselves, the hospital was able to charge about half the regular hospital rate. The teaching unit was the only one of its kind in the country and placed a heavy emphasis on teaching diabetics to care for themselves, since education was a key to survival.

In 1958, Lahey physicians Herb Adams and Elton Watkins, Jr., successfully carried out an autologous transplant of parathyroid glands in a Deaconess patient and received worldwide publicity. The following year, on the basis of work carried out by Jim Tullis and Hugh Pyle, the Deaconess became the first hospital in the world to have a bank of blood platelets ready for immediate transfusion, as well as a bank of frozen blood cells for long-term storage.

In the early 1960s, Elton Watkins and Robert D. Sullivan of the Lahey Clinic directed an early chemotherapy program for cancer patients and developed a portable pump for treatment on an outpatient basis. Later in the decade, Joseph Crehan, a Deaconess anesthesiologist, developed a Respiratory Therapy and Equipment Service at the hospital which prepared and followed patients pre- and postoperatively, considerably reducing the mortality and morbidity associated with pulmonary complications. The unit became a model for training respiratory therapists nationwide.

In 1966, under the direction of O. Stevens Leland, a coronary care unit was opened to provide close monitoring of patients with heart irregularities. The nation's first Stoma Rehabilitation Clinic was organized by Deaconess surgeon John L. Rowbotham. Created with the assistance of federal funding, its purpose was to instruct patients with ileostomies, colostomies, or ileal bladders on how to live with their stomas. The clinic, which accepted patients from any doctor in New England, was concerned not only with the care of the stoma and the use of various appliances, but also with patients' emotional and social adjustment.

In 1970, surgeons Wilford Neptune and Anthony P. Monaco performed simultaneous open-heart surgery and a kidney transplant on a young woman who not only survived, but went on to lead a normal life. The procedures were considered surgical feats at the time because of their intricacies and simultaneity.

It is important to remember that all of these innovations took place in a hospital that was dominated by private practitioners and their patients, many of whom had been referred to one of the clinics or to independent members of the staff because of their specialized skills and clinical abilities and reputations, not because of their renown for research or teaching. Many Deaconess doctors were known for making twice-daily rounds and for carefully shielding their patients from residents. Some floors had residents; others did not. Contact with private patients by medical students was very limited.

As time passed, although the Deaconess was home to more research and teaching than formerly, it was still not primarily a teaching or research institution. Nor was it a community hospital in the usual sense of that term: it did not secure admittances through a busy emergency room. A four-bed observation unit was opened in 1967, a kind of substitute for an emergency room, mainly used by patients of staff doctors, not by the general public. The facility was needed in order to satisfy the training requirements for certification of the house officer training programs.

The hospital's medical, nursing, and lay leadership alike agreed that what made the Deaconess stand out was its patient care, about whose excellence they were not reluctant to preach, both internally and externally. In periodic orientation sessions for new employees held in the Joslin Auditorium, Lowry discussed the hospital's history and philosophy and stressed the primacy of patient care. Each patient, he told new staff, was an individual — he entreated them never to refer to "that appendectomy down in 402." The same sentiment appeared in large print on the first page of the hospital's seventy-fifth anniversary commemorative booklet, "The essence of the Deaconess, concerned and compassionate patient care, are timeless characteristics of a fine institution."

A DERAILED MERGER

During the 1960s, while the Deaconess was devoting funds and energy to physical expansion and increasing teaching and research endeavors, the Lahey Clinic, under McLean and Adams, was concerned with long-term planning. The Lahey Clinic, which had continued to grow during the 1950s and 1960s, found itself cramped for space in its Kenmore Square location. Equally important, the clinic concluded that its own future depended on the availability of many more hospital beds than it controlled at the time.

While both fostering and participating in the Deaconess's expansion, Lahey Clinic's management entered into a long courtship of New

England Baptist Hospital, its other primary facility, with a view to relocating its Kenmore Square headquarters and diagnostic center in proximity to the Baptist on Boston's Mission Hill. The Baptist, in Adams's view, merely strung the Lahey along over a period of years. Then, in November 1969, the Baptist announced plans to build, essentially on its own, a new 300-bed hospital complex. Not long after that, the Baptist rejected the Lahey's formal proposal of a merger. Its affections spurned, the clinic subsequently pursued other options, including acquiring a site in Boston or Watertown or building an entirely new hospital in suburban Westwood, though significant problems developed with each of these possibilities.

It is not surprising, therefore, that the clinic also approached Deaconess management in 1970 about a possible merger. Nor is it astonishing that Lowry and the Deaconess trustee Executive Committee were willing to consider the proposal. At the time the Lahey Clinic had claims on 40 percent of the hospital's private beds; the Joslin Clinic was allocated 25 percent; and the general staff, 35 percent. In 1971, the Lahey Clinic had 84 doctors on the Deaconess staff; the Joslin Clinic, 15; the Overholt Clinic, 4; and there were 119 physicians unaffiliated with any of the clinics. In addition, the Lahey Clinic accounted for a disproportionate number of surgical admissions. In seven specialties of medicine and surgery, the Lahey was responsible for more than 45 percent of patient days and constituted at least half of the Deaconess's total staff in those specialties: cardiology, gastroenterology, neurology, neurosurgery, orthopedic surgery, psychiatry, and urology.

It was clear to the hospital administration that if the Lahey Clinic were to go elsewhere or to build elsewhere, it would result in huge losses of patients and staff from the Deaconess. The clinic's departure would threaten several of the hospital's residency programs and also would not bode well for the Deaconess's reputation. One of the most highly regarded specialty clinics in the country, the Lahey encouraged its doctors to publish papers in medical journals. In these years Lahey Clinic doctors published many more scholarly papers than others on the Deaconess staff.

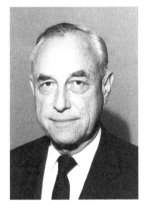

DR. HERBERT DAN ADAMS, CA. 1970. *Adams first came to the Deaconess as a medical student and was appointed a Lahey surgical fellow in 1930. He joined the Lahey Clinic staff in 1936 and eventually headed the clinic from 1962 to 1969.*

Concerns about a Lahey departure were heightened by a strong perception among the hospital's management that the general staff was aging and was not replenishing itself sufficiently. That failure was partly attributable to the changing economics and practice of medicine, and partly to the limited supply of beds. Members of the general staff had not been eager to increase their own numbers since that would only have increased competition for a scarce resource — beds.

Further, the Lahey Clinic commanded respect within the Deaconess Executive Committee because of the belief that it practiced the best medicine in the hospital and accounted for a majority of its most difficult cases. A merger with the Lahey Clinic was also attractive because it might end infighting and unify the staff; it held out promise, as well, of facilitating fund raising and expansion, possibly out of the city, perhaps through the establishment of a satellite hospital, or even complete relocation. The Longwood medical area was cramped, and traffic congestion, crime, and social unrest were growing. The expanding, more affluent suburbs beckoned, attracting individuals and institutions alike looking to escape the city's problems.

To Neil Sedgwick, who had first suggested the idea to Don Lowry, a merger seemed a natural consequence since the Deaconess knew all about running a hospital and the Lahey Clinic knew all about operating a group practice. High-level representatives of both institutions began to meet quietly in 1970 and 1971 to discuss a possible merger or consolidation. The discussions were kept secret because of the expectation that such a move would be controversial.

Various components of the hospital were represented at these deliberations, though in small numbers, including Alex Marble and Bob Bradley of the Joslin Clinic, Lyman Hoyt of the independent staff, Bill Meissner, and Laurie MacLure and Vince Vappi from the trustees. The Lahey Clinic was represented by John Norcross, who succeeded Adams, and by Sedgwick and McLean. Lowry and the Executive Committee also brought in John Glover and the Cambridge Research Institute, who had been hired as consultants in 1970 to help think through long-term planning.

Most doctors at both institutions were not told about the discussions. Lowry deliberately kept Tullis in the dark because he wanted to shield him from the wrath of the independent medical staff, many of whom had not been keen on having a chief of medicine in the first place. Indeed, Tullis first heard of the merger when MacLure called him one day and asked him to come over to Dean Ebert's office at the medical school for the announcement of a merger between the hospital and the Lahey Clinic. Tullis could hardly believe his ears — he realized that if he had not been aware of this merger, very few other doctors could have known either. Ebert's imprimatur suggested that the old animosity between Harvard and the Lahey Clinic had dissipated. In fact, by this time quite a few Lahey physicians and surgeons held clinical appointments at Harvard, a relationship that Frank Lahey had never allowed during his lifetime.

In early September 1971, the Deaconess Executive Committee unanimously recommended to the full board of trustees a consolidation with the Lahey Clinic. The committee also asked for authorization to proceed with discussions aimed at effectuating the merger. Within hours after these recommendations had been disclosed, however, an agitated general staff began to organize meetings in opposition. Although the independents were all going to be "grandfathered" in, they nevertheless were frightened by the prospect of a Lahey takeover. All the traditional disdain by independent physicians toward "corporate medicine" and group practice came rushing to the fore.

Many independent doctors were angry at Lowry, in part because he had kept them uninformed. One leading insurgent, who had been Lowry's friend for many years, said he would never trust him again. At one meeting, doctors discussed getting rid of Lowry; this angered and dismayed Bill Meissner who knew that Lowry had only been trying to do what was best for the hospital. Given the strength of feeling against the merger, it may be speculated that early disclosure or greater inclusiveness would not have made much of a difference in the doctors' reaction.

As it happened, many independent staff members had hospital trustees as patients and in many cases they had been their patients for a long time. These doctors quickly organized a series of visits, often going in pairs to see individual patient-trustees, including some members of the Executive Committee itself, at their homes at night. These "house calls" proved highly effective. Although the Executive

Committee had voted unanimously in favor of a merger, it soon became evident that the idea did not command a majority of the fifty-one trustees. Consequently, within two weeks of approving the merger in principle, the Executive Committee reversed itself and decided to defer action.

The Executive Committee referred the merger report for further study to an ad hoc committee to be appointed by the president. The group was to be broadly representative of all segments of the hospital, and it was asked to consider other alternatives to those contained in the merger report. In fact, no such committee was ever appointed, recalled Lowry, though the matter was discussed by the long-range planning panel.

Although the merger idea continued to appeal to certain individuals, including even some independents, it was dead for all intents and purposes. Opposed to it were not only most members of the general staff, including Jim Tullis, but most of the Joslin Clinic, whose staff members and trustees worried that their own clinic would lose its identity if it were swallowed up. Moreover, the Joslin was moving increasingly into research and into a close affiliation with Harvard. It was hard to see how that would fit into the Lahey Clinic's developing interest in relocating to the suburbs.

By June 1972, Vince Vappi reported to the Executive Committee that there was too much opposition to a merger among the independent and Joslin staffs for the idea to be given any further consideration. But what would the Deaconess do when Lahey left, which, in the absence of a merger, now seemed virtually inevitable? How would it fill the 40 percent of private beds accounted for by the Lahey and for the commensurate gaps in staffing? How would it make up for the loss in reputation that would surely follow?

The hospital's Long-Range Planning Committee grappled with these questions and reached three general conclusions: "(1) that the future of the New England Deaconess Hospital [lay] in the area of a specialty-referral hospital, (2) that it [would] require a gradually increasing interaction and/or affiliation with a medical school, and (3) that there [would] be need for some form of a more cohesive organization of the independent medical staff as may be necessary to react to the Deaconess Hospital in the future without the Lahey Clinic and in order to meet the evolving needs imposed on us by society at large." These conclusions, it should be emphasized, were general in nature. It remained to be seen how the Deaconess would deal with the Lahey Clinic's eventual departure.

By mid-1972, despite its rich history, healthy finances, accomplished staff, and full beds, the Deaconess faced a more uncertain future than at any time since its early years.

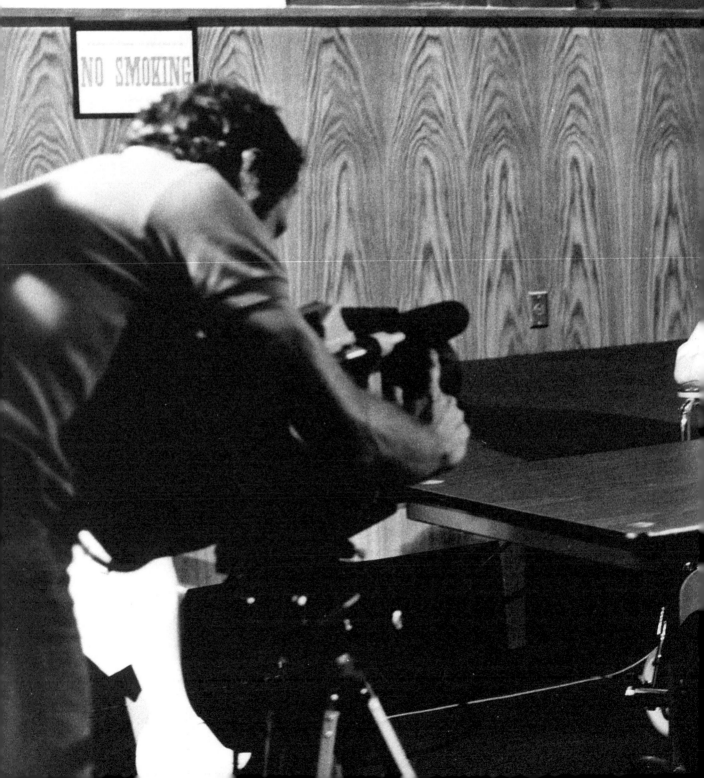

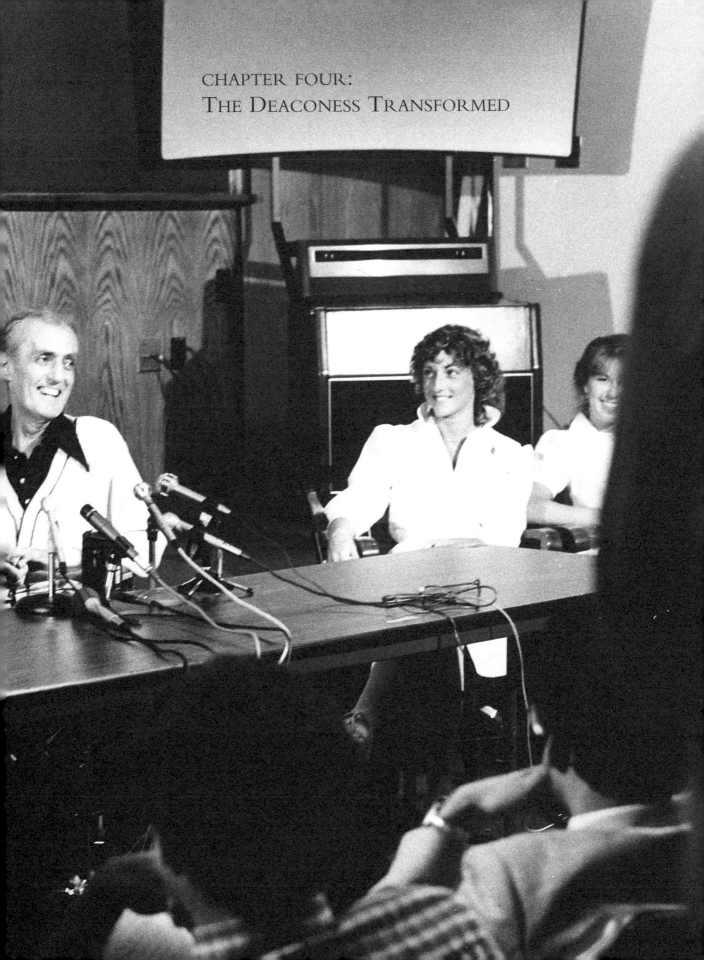

CHAPTER FOUR:
THE DEACONESS TRANSFORMED

CHAPTER FOUR:
THE DEACONESS TRANSFORMED

The lay and medical leadership of New England Deaconess Hospital made far-reaching decisions in the early and mid-1970s which laid the foundation for the hospital's future as an academic and tertiary-care institution. As these strategies were being formulated and implemented, the hospital altered its governing structure and effectuated a management transition. During the succeeding decade, the Deaconess augmented its professional staff, appointed new department chiefs, installed modern technologies, expanded and improved residency programs, and completed several construction projects. By early 1985 a metamorphosis was evident in the hospital's purpose and direction.

A FOUNDATION FOR THE FUTURE

Following the denouement of the Lahey merger, the Deaconess's Long-Range Planning Committee became a sounding board for ideas about the hospital's future. The group was led by Marvin G. Schorr, a trustee and Executive Committee member. With key doctors, administrators, and trustees as members, the committee was broadly representative of constituencies within the hospital. (In 1973 Vincent Vappi became president of the Deaconess board and Laurens MacLure moved up to the chairmanship, succeeding Francis Capper, who had retired after a remarkable forty-one-year association with the hospital.) Schorr had been recruited to the Deaconess board in 1971 by Vince Vappi and Colby Hewitt, Jr. Schorr and Vappi, who were old and close friends, also became business partners when their companies merged in 1972.

Trained as a physicist in the 1950s, with three other scientists Schorr had helped establish Technical Operations, Inc., a contract research company. He served as its business leader and the company thrived. Schorr was favorably impressed by the doctors he met at the Deaconess, including Jim Tullis and Neil Sedgwick, and he quickly became enthralled with the hospital and its work. He enjoyed wrestling with the complex issues which the Deaconess faced in the early 1970s. Analytical, dispassionate, and tactful, Schorr had the necessary attributes to help formulate a long-range plan for an institution in which there were honest and strongly felt differences of opinion.

The Long-Range Planning Committee authorized a study by the Cambridge Research Institute to examine trends in the hospital industry

and the Deaconess's position in the Boston area. The consultants presented
a number of options for the hospital's future, including: (1) becoming a
community hospital; (2) remaining a specialty-referral hospital while strengthening ties to Harvard Medical School; or (3) moving toward a contractual
relationship with a health maintenance organization (HMO) or even
forming the nucleus of an HMO. Two of the three proposals were rejected
as unworkable. Evolving into a community hospital was not a promising
position for the Deaconess since both Beth Israel and the Peter Bent
Brigham were fulfilling that role already in the Longwood section of Boston
and out toward Brookline and nearby suburbs. The position would also
require major changes in the kinds of services the Deaconess offered and the
number and type of personnel it employed. Similarly, health maintenance
organizations were still too experimental and such a move would entail
significant risk for the Deaconess: HMOs depended on primary-care physicians, not the legion of specialists who constituted the vast majority of
the Deaconess staff.

The second of the three options was the most plausible; indeed,
it was closest to the role the Deaconess already played. Strengthening
the hospital's position as a specialty-referral facility while moving closer
to Harvard thus became the underlying strategy of Deaconess management.
But implementation of this course would require significant augmentation
of the hospital's staff and an expansion of the referral base in anticipation
of the Lahey Clinic's departure. A closer relationship with Harvard, however,
would threaten doctors' customary autonomy. And although the hospital's
key trustees were certain about the direction they believed the hospital needed
to traverse over the long term, that did not mean that the hospital's staff
was prepared to take concrete steps to get there in the short term, as the
response to a proposal put forth by Jim Tullis in June 1972 made clear.

Although Tullis had disapproved of the Lahey merger, he
understood that the idea had appealed to certain trustees because it assured the
hospital of a dynamic and high-quality medical staff. The union would have
solved the problem of an aging independent staff that was not replenishing
itself and that had resisted adding significantly to its ranks. Tullis argued in his
proposal that it was in the nature of a clinic or group practice to want to grow,
while the opposite was true of independent practitioners. "Any physician
in independent practice invariably will attempt to protect his personal interests

and keep competition in his field to the minimum, commensurate with his time and ability to render service. If he did not, he would be stupid," Tullis wrote with characteristic directness.

Tullis suggested that "Deaconess Hospital itself practice medicine." In fact, he pointed out, it was already doing so, a reality not widely acknowledged. At the time, twenty members of the active staff in medicine and surgery were receiving a monthly payroll check from the hospital for services rendered, which were mostly administrative, but which also involved some direct patient care. In addition, another twenty or so members of the pathology and radiology staffs drew hospital salaries. Indeed, Shields Warren and Bill Meissner's success in building the Department of Pathology with a full-time staff partially inspired Tullis in his plan.

Tullis recommended to the Deaconess Corporation that a new professional division be established. Its members would be full time and would receive salaries and benefits from the hospital. Tullis antici-pated that this division would create a financial surplus, allowing the hospital to recruit and support young physicians "whom we need and currently cannot afford." Tullis also wanted to increase the power of department chairmen to recruit new staff members to the hospital, which implied a commensurate reduction in the influence of the Long-Range Planning Committee on staff membership.

The "Tullis proposal" became the focal point for an internal debate that raged for more than two years involving the Long-Range Planning Committee, the Executive Committee of the trustees, and the medical staff. For many doctors, both independents and members of the clinics alike, the proposal represented an undesirable turn in the direction of an academic institution such as the Peter Bent Brigham. "The one thing we never want to become is another Peter Bent Brigham Hospital," Don Lowry recalled doctors telling him repeatedly.

These physicians feared what sometimes followed when academicians took over a hospital and installed powerful department heads — incumbent staff members were forced out as patient care took second place to teaching and research. Deaconess doctors worried that a new full-time, hospital-based group practice would receive preferential treatment; that, in turn, they believed would translate into diminished

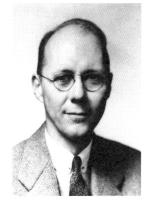

DR. JAMES L. TULLIS, CA. 1960. *An important figure in the transformation of Deaconess Hospital from a fine tertiary-care facility to an important academic and research center, Tullis became chief of medicine in 1964. His proposal for reorganizing the hospital's medical staff was adopted in 1974, laying the groundwork for the modern Deaconess Hospital.*

access for themselves and their clinics. Doctors from the Lahey Clinic participated in these discussions even though in 1971 the clinic had purchased a large new site in Burlington. However, it would be several years before the Lahey won the necessary approvals to build a 200-bed medical center there; from 1972 to 1974 the Lahey Clinic remained a player in discussions about the Deaconess's future, although a diminishing one as its departure became more certain.

"Full time" also meant that limitations would be set on individual doctors' earnings, as they were at Harvard Medical School — indeed, Tullis used Harvard as a model for his proposal. Although it was generally considered crass to talk openly about money, there was no doubt in the minds of the hospital's lay and medical leadership that economic interests were a central underlying concern to the doctors, probably *the* central underlying concern, noble words about patient care notwithstanding. "You're not going to institutionalize me, Jim," one prominent doctor bluntly told Tullis. "I'm going to take all of the money out of the practice of medicine that I can."

The Tullis proposal was scrutinized, praised, condemned, and refined, while its author suffered a certain amount of resentment from the staff. Tullis could later recall with wry amusement how the doctors' conference room in the cafeteria would empty out when he entered. To be sure, many doctors who disagreed with Tullis maintained their admiration and respect for him; even his detractors conceded his brilliance, and there were a number of staff members who tacitly or openly agreed with his diagnosis and prescription for the hospital. Albert I. (Ivy) DeFriez, for example, an outstanding general internist whom Tullis had recruited to the staff, was one who spoke out in support of the plan.

Nonetheless, in the spring of 1974, 103 doctors, including members of the three clinics — Lahey, Joslin, and Overholt — constituting somewhat less than half of the hospital's total staff, signed a petition opposing "the development of a 'full-time,' hospital-based group practice. We find the results of such undertakings at nearby teaching hospitals to be disruptive, particularly the creation of preferential access to hospital facilities." In May, C. Burns Roehrig, an internist who was then chairman of the hospital's Medical Administrative Board, addressed a special meeting of the Deaconess Board of Trustees. In a moderate tone, he urged caution upon them and extolled the kind of personalized care offered by individual physicians. He quoted the medical staff's bylaws which "recognize the ultimate authority of the Trustees in the guidance and management of the Deaconess as a corporate structure." Roehrig concluded, "We *must* and we *will* find a way into the future for this institution in which the Medical Staff *can* still *work together!*"

  In contrast to what had occurred following the announcement of the Lahey merger, the Executive Committee did not capitulate this time. The planning process and the debate had been both protracted and open. Therefore, complaints about a closed and secretive process were not credible, although some continued to be voiced nevertheless. No one, however, had come up with an effective alternative to Tullis's proposal. Recent court decisions had expanded the legal responsibility of trustees to include the quality and efficiency of medical care. At the same time, hospitals were under increasing regulatory pressures and restraints. Deaconess trustees had a fiduciary responsibility for the welfare of the institution as a whole and felt that in order to maintain the hospital's viability, they had to be prepared to move with the times.

  Many of the objections and objectors to the Tullis plan appeared parochial and self-interested to the hospital's lay management and trustees and to its medical leadership as well. Indeed, in 1973, when William V. McDermott, Jr., director of the Harvard Surgical Service at Boston City Hospital, was contemplating moving to the Deaconess, he described the hospital to its trustees as "the best medical condominium in Boston." His observation, which was a way of saying that the hospital lacked unity, rang true with many trustees, though this comment was not well received by the staff. Proponents of the Tullis plan occupied higher moral ground; at a meeting of the Medical Administrative Board, Tullis emphasized that the proposal had been written with just one thing in mind — Deaconess Hospital, not the individual interests of any group.

  Finally, the Tullis proposal was actually modest in scope and did not threaten people immediately. As Tullis himself repeatedly pointed out, the Deaconess already had a good number of part- and full-time doctors. At a critical moment in the debate, Tullis somewhat mollified the general internists by agreeing that he would not take any general internists into Deaconess Medicine, except for doctors who worked in the clinic for hospital employees. He pledged to hire only subspecialists.

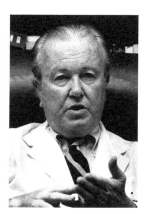

Dr. William V. McDermott, Jr., ca. 1975. The David W. and David Cheever Professor of Surgery at Harvard, McDermott brought the Fifth Harvard Surgical Service from Boston City Hospital to the Deaconess in 1973. A well-known specialist in biliary and gastrointestinal disorders, McDermott directed the Department of Surgery's residency and research activities. Following Sedgwick's retirement, McDermott assumed all duties as chairman of Deaconess surgery.

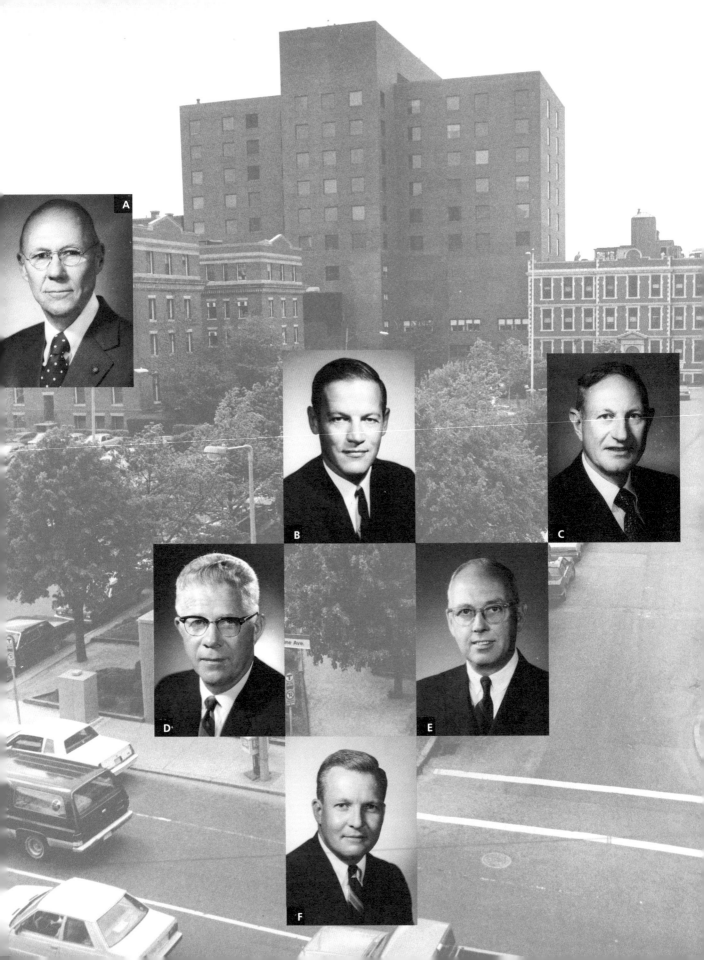

Despite these concessions, in September 1974, a majority of the Medical Administrative Board voted for a resolution recommending to the trustees' Executive Committee that the Tullis proposal be tabled for an extended period of time. Yet the same group simultaneously passed a resolution praising Tullis for his hard work.

A month later the Executive Committee *appeared* to concede when it agreed that it would be inadvisable "at this time to implement a formally structured clinical group practice in the hospital." However, it reaffirmed the goals set by the Long-Range Planning Committee, gave Tullis a renewed vote of confidence as head of the Department of Medicine, and, most important, asked him to assume the position full time, thus approving a practice plan in principle. The committee also asked Lowry to continue exploring "various means of structuring this program in a way that is financially sound and most acceptable to all the hospital's constituencies." Thus, the camel's nose went under the tent.

AT THE END OF 1974, Tullis donated his practice "lock, stock, and barrel" to the hospital and became a full-time Deaconess employee. Going full time was a personal sacrifice. "As one who has now done it," Tullis reported two months later, "I can only say I did so with [a] certain sadness." It meant both a loss of income and a loss of independence. He continued, "I can't tell you the startled amusement I felt when I went away recently for a week in Nassau and was asked the afternoon before leaving if this was a vacation week I was taking or a professional trip! It was not a professional trip. But that's the first time since I was in prep school forty-three years ago that it has been anybody's business except my own where I was going or for what purpose, and it is the first time anyone cared." One thing that had not changed, however, was his level of effort. He was still working sixty to seventy hours a week — "I'm too old a dog to learn new tricks," he remarked.

As expected, only a small number of subspecialists from the Department of Medicine joined Tullis initially in what was called Deaconess Medicine — Murray Bern, his assistant in hematology/ oncology, and Chief of Cardiology O. Stevens Leland and his two assistants, Robert W. Healy and Samuel J. Shubrooks, Jr. A fourth cardiologist, Ahmed Mohiuddin, elected to be part time, while a fifth,

Harold D. Levine, remained fully independent. Tullis pointed out that Levine was "strictly a clinical cardiologist who only wants to see patients. He doesn't want to learn catheter techniques or perform echograms, nor does he wish to administer teaching programs or supervise house officers in a CCU. To me, he is the epitome of the bedside clinician, whom we must cherish and protect here at the Deaconess."

Leland had come out of an academic background at Boston City Hospital and Harvard Medical School. Since his recruitment by Tullis in 1965, he had increasingly become involved in administering sophisticated new procedures that were emerging in these years. He felt a little uncomfortable personally receiving the lucrative fees that cardiology was beginning to generate and was strongly committed to teaching. He had built up a fellowship program in cardiology in addition to running the cardiac catheterization laboratory. Although going full time involved a personal financial sacrifice, Leland did not give it much thought. In view of his own values, Tullis's leadership, and the hospital's needs, "it just seemed the right thing to do," he recalled. Leland's change to full-time status, like that of Tullis, was not applauded by some of the staff, who regarded him as a turncoat. In time, the cardiology division generated healthy surpluses, which the hospital used to recruit and support young subspecialists in other areas, just as Tullis had predicted.

TULLIS OFFERED HIS REORGANIZATION PLAN IN 1972 and it was formally adopted two years later. In the meantime, in 1973, the Deaconess seized a chance to upgrade dramatically its academic status in surgery. The opportunity arose when financial and political considerations converged to squeeze Harvard and Tufts medical schools out of Boston City Hospital; Mayor Kevin H. White handed the municipal hospital's training programs over to Boston University exclusively. This development marked a sharp break with history: Harvard's association with Boston City had begun with the hospital's establishment in 1864, when David William Cheever of Harvard became its first chief of surgery.

In 1973 William V. McDermott, the David W. and David Cheever Professor of Surgery at Harvard, was the director of the Harvard Surgical Service at Boston City Hospital, formerly and often still known as the Fifth Harvard Surgical Service. A well-known professor of surgery, particularly through his work on the liver and with gastrointestinal disorders, McDermott found himself in the unusual and somewhat awkward position of being a chaired professor of surgery at Harvard who, through no fault of his own, had lost his hospital base of operations. Meanwhile, many in the Deaconess's upper lay and medical ranks — Lowry, MacLure, Schorr, Vappi, and Meissner, Sedgwick, and Tullis — had concluded that the hospital's future lay in moving closer to Harvard and in becoming more academically oriented, though they avoided saying so too loudly because of the concept's lack of popularity with significant parts of the medical staff. With the support of key trustees and doctors, Lowry initiated discussions with McDermott and Harvard Medical School.

It was understood that bringing McDermott to the Deaconess would effectively give the Department of Surgery full status at Harvard instantaneously; under the Harvard system, McDermott, as a full, tenured professor in the academic faculty, had considerable authority in recommending appointments to Harvard's clinical faculty. His move to the Deaconess promised to strengthen the hospital's surgical residency program. McDermott had previously rotated residents from the program at Boston City to the Deaconess; now the Fifth Harvard Surgical Service itself, which in 1973 had forty residents, would be based at the Deaconess, while residents rotated to a number of other hospitals to round out their training. Hospitals, it should be noted, not Harvard Medical School itself, ran *graduate* training programs, but having a Harvard professor based at the Deaconess would unquestionably enhance the hospital's stature in the academic community.

Harvard's Dean Robert Ebert was pleased at the prospect of McDermott's finding a home at the Deaconess. Contrary to what some people might have thought, Ebert had a low-key position about the Deaconess and was not trying to "colonize" it for Harvard. Although the Deaconess was conveniently located near the medical school, which added to its attractiveness, Harvard did not suffer from a shortage of hospitals in which to train students, even without Boston City. The Deaconess was known to Ebert as a fine private hospital offering excellent patient care, but it was hardly alone in either of these respects. From Ebert's perspective the Deaconess affiliation with the Joslin Clinic, which had a close connection to Harvard, was actually more important.

A number of independent surgeons at the Deaconess were distinctly unhappy about McDermott's impending arrival. Neither McDermott nor the other academic surgeons he brought with him had large private practices, certainly not compared with those of the independent staff or of the Overholt Clinic. Nevertheless, some independent surgeons worried that they might somehow have less access to operating rooms. Ironically, they also were concerned that academic surgeons did not perform *enough* surgery to be as proficient as they should be. In addition, the fear remained that patient care would devolve to residents once academic surgeons arrived on the scene. Despite some unhappiness and grumbling among the private surgeons, Neil Sedgwick, who was chairman of surgery and would remain so after McDermott's arrival, fully supported McDermott's move to the Deaconess. Marv Schorr later reflected that Sedgwick's statesmanship in this matter probably saved the hospital a great deal of internal strife.

Sedgwick and McDermott liked and respected one another; they were both gentlemen and were self-confident and unthreatened by the other's presence. Although it was unusual for a full professor of surgery not to be chief of surgery in the hospital at which he was based, McDermott accepted the situation. Nor did it concern Sedgwick that McDermott, not he, was a chaired professor at Harvard. (Sedgwick was later promoted to a clinical professorship.) Indeed, Sedgwick understood that if the hospital were to move closer to Harvard and strengthen its residency program further, it made good sense to have McDermott there. McDermott's presence could, for example, enhance the hospital's reputation among Harvard medical students, some of whom McDermott and his associates taught, making them more likely to apply for residencies at the Deaconess.

In 1973, McDermott joined the Deaconess staff. From the beginning Sedgwick and McDermott worked well together, complementing each other's skills. As chairman, Sedgwick ran the operating rooms and the ICUs, with all that this responsibility entailed, while McDermott assumed responsibility for the residency program, research activities, and Harvard relationships. John V. Pikula, a general surgeon who initially came with McDermott from Boston City, assisted with internship and residency training programs. McDermott advised Sedgwick on departmental structure and staffing and McDermott helped recruit a number of outstanding surgeons, probably none more so than Daniel Miller, a specialist in head and neck surgery, who relocated from Massachusetts Eye and Ear Infirmary.

To be sure, outstanding surgeons were at the Deaconess before McDermott relocated there, among them Mian Ashraf, Blake Cady, F. Henry Ellis, Charles Fager, Carl Hoar, Wilford Neptune, John Rowbotham, George Starkey, Elton Watkins, Frank Wheelock, Francis Wolfort, and Clement Yahia — all of whom were either independents or affiliated with the Lahey and Overholt clinics.

Sedgwick, an outstanding teacher of residents as well as a busy and superb surgeon, continued to play a vital teaching role. In addition to having outstanding technique, Sedgwick was an extremely fast surgeon. He taught through a kind of preceptor system, which was very popular with residents, and he took a great personal interest in his protégés.

McDermott became director of the Cancer Research Institute, which was controlled by the Deaconess, not Harvard. He formally received this appointment in February of 1974, seven months after his move to the Deaconess. The CRI position had opened up when its previous occupant, the likable and talented George Nichols, stepped down. McDermott brought new vitality to CRI, while reassuring its researchers that their positions were secure.

Following the transfer of grants from the Sears Surgical Laboratory at Boston City, a number of talented physician-researchers came to CRI, including Anthony Monaco, an associate professor of surgery at Harvard, and George Blackburn, an assistant professor of surgery. At CRI Monaco directed the Division of Transplantation and Immunology, in which researcher Takashi Maki played a major role, while Blackburn headed the Division of Nutrition, which became an important interdisciplinary program with the presence of Bruce Bistrian from the Department of Medicine. In 1980, after a new wing was added to CRI, George H. A. Clowes, Jr., relocated from Boston City to head the research effort of the Division on Metabolism in Shock and Trauma. By historical coincidence, Clowes's father had played a central role in the initial production of insulin by Eli Lilly and Company. The first dose of insulin available in New England (supplied by the Lilly Company) had been administered by Howard Root at Deaconess Hospital a half century before.

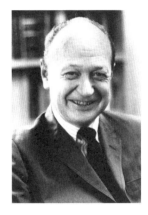

DR. ROBERT H. EBERT, 1968. As dean of Harvard Medical School, Ebert was instrumental in the hospital's early efforts to join the family of Harvard teaching institutions. His flexible and diplomatic approach with the Deaconess leadership was an important factor in negotiations between the medical school and the hospital.

CHANGES IN GOVERNANCE AND LEADERSHIP

By 1973 and 1974, in the midst of the debate over the hospital's future, important changes were also occurring in governance and management. Overseeing the Deaconess in 1973 were nearly 200 corporators who met annually and were comparable to stockholders in a corporation. The corporators elected a Board of Trustees that numbered fifty-one, which, under the bylaws, was ceded a great deal of authority by the corporation. The Board of Trustees, which met quarterly, in turn delegated day-to-day oversight to a thirteen-member Executive Committee, which met monthly.

In 1973 two doctors, Charles Fager of the Lahey Clinic and C. Burns Roehrig, who was at the time president of the Medical Administrative Board, and Dick Lee, the hospital's chief operating officer, were *ex officio* members of the Executive Committee. Don Lowry, who was executive vice president — in effect, the hospital's chief executive officer — and a trustee, was a regular member, as were Laurens MacLure, who was chairman of the board, and Vince Vappi, who was president of the corporation.

Partly because of what had happened after the proposed merger with the Lahey Clinic, when individual doctors lobbied trustees successfully against the union, members of the Executive Committee saw a need to change the way the hospital was governed. They felt that trustees deferred to doctors and were not sufficiently informed or involved to guide the hospital successfully into the future. MacLure, Schorr, Vappi, and other Executive Committee members realized that with the new direction the hospital was taking, they would need trustees who would be more concerned with larger institutional issues and less susceptible to their own doctors' powers of persuasion. The hospital needed its medical staff, but trustees had to put the hospital's overarching interests first.

Consequently, in the spring of 1974, the Executive Committee appointed an ad hoc committee chaired by attorney William B. Tyler to review governance. Following a year of study, the committee recommended that the Board of Trustees be reduced to twenty-one members over a five-year period and that it meet monthly. The Board of Trustees would in effect become the Executive Committee, which itself would assume a secondary role, acting only in emergencies. The committee also advised that the medical staff, through election, have representation on the board, assuring it a voice. These recommendations were accepted and new bylaws were approved by the corporation at a special meeting in the fall of 1975. In ensuing years, the new structure worked appreciably better than the old, allowing those governing the hospital to act in a more unified way. One of the first doctors elected to the board was Sedgwick, an ironic vote in view of his close association with the unpopular Lahey merger. His election indicated the unusually high regard in which he was held.

Meanwhile, the Executive Committee also had to look for a successor to Don Lowry, who wanted to retire; he would turn sixty-two in 1975. Indeed, he had informed the committee of his desire in 1973, but the group had been slow to act, perhaps because so much else was happening and because it was difficult to contemplate the Deaconess without Lowry, the hospital's strong leader for two decades. After a year passed and nothing seemed to be happening in the search for a successor, Lowry became more insistent about retirement, and a search committee, chaired by Marv Schorr, was established.

It was a turbulent and uncertain time in the hospital's history and the committee discussed the sort of person it would need in the years ahead. First, the new leader would need to be a conciliator, not a confrontationist, who would move the staff gradually in the direction of Harvard and academia. It would also require someone with stature in the broader community, one who could negotiate with Harvard and with other hospitals and who could recruit new trustees with management know-how and wealth. And it would need someone with financial acumen since it was becoming clear that hospitals were entering a more competitive and demanding economic environment.

Jim Tullis has recalled that he was playing golf with Laurie MacLure one day and MacLure, who as chairman of the hospital board had appointed the search committee, asked him when it was going to come up with a recommendation for Lowry's successor. Tullis indicated that he had a very good candidate in mind but that he probably would not take the job. "Who's that?" MacLure asked. "You," Tullis replied. "Me? I'm a banker," MacLure remarked incredulously. He was then senior vice president of The Boston Company. Tullis argued that

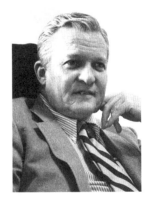

LAURENS MACLURE, CA. 1977. *Through three decades of service to the hospital, MacLure held a number of leadership positions including chairman of the board. In 1975 he succeeded Robert D. Lowry as the hospital's chief executive and served until 1989.*

hospitals were going to need top financial management over the next ten years and he asked whether MacLure would take the job. MacLure said that if the committee desired, he would consider the offer.

Next Vince Vappi approached MacLure with the idea of taking the position. Once MacLure indicated his willingness, the search was effectively over. MacLure, who was actually getting ready to leave the board, had risen up through the volunteer ranks over the course of nearly twenty years, having been assistant treasurer, vice president, president, and, for the previous three years, chairman. MacLure was familiar with all of the Deaconess's central issues and all of its key actors. Had there been overt opposition, he recalled, he would not have agreed to accept the job, but both the hospital's medical leaders and the trustees encouraged him to take it.

MacLure asked that in becoming chief executive officer, he be given the title of president, instead of executive vice president, which had been Lowry's designation since 1967. The Executive Committee readily agreed. This change, which was in line with a national trend although ahead of most other Boston institutions, reflected the contemporary notion that hospitals were more like businesses, which needed modern management to deal with a dynamic world, and less the voluntary, charitable organizations of old, which were simply administered in rather routine fashion.

Indeed, Medicare, by insuring all of the nation's elderly, had made it more profitable to go into the hospital business and thus had helped to usher in investor-owned hospital chains while also blurring the distinction between nonprofit and for-profit institutions, whose financing and behavior were more similar than not. Hospitals were becoming a big business and they were a growth area — in the mid-1970s, hospitals were the fastest growing industry in the United States, outpacing computers, electronics, and soft drinks. The fact that MacLure came from the business world reflected these new perceptions and realities.

On June 1, 1975, MacLure became a full-time employee of the Deaconess while Lowry stayed on until November of that year to assist with the transition. Upon Lowry's retirement, the trustees renamed the medical office facility which he had been so instrumental in erecting the R. D. Lowry Medical Office Building. Dick Lee stayed on as director and chief operating officer. Although there were disparities in philosophy and style between MacLure and Lee, Lee did an effective job operationally while supporting MacLure's overall strategy.

MacLure proved to be the right person for the time. His stature, self-confidence, and interpersonal skills, along with his financial, managerial, and negotiating abilities, served the hospital well. He recruited a new generation of successful business people to the board and represented the hospital effectively with Harvard. As an active participant in the long-range planning process, MacLure firmly believed that the hospital's future lay with Harvard, positioned as a specialty-referral hospital, able to recruit a first-class medical and surgical staff. But MacLure also appreciated the political risks of articulating these goals either too loudly or too often. He had a reassuring style and was a consensus-builder; he was tactful but also tenacious in moving the process forward. "My strategy was *never* have a battle — avoid confrontation," he later reflected. "You knew what the goal was and you just kept plugging away and if you got stopped on Route 1, you went over to Route 2, took a secondary road. And if that was blockaded, try Route 3. You just kept moving the troops and if you could move on the western front, you moved there and if that was blocked you tried to move on the eastern front."

GROWTH AND REGULATION

Don Lowry, of course, had been a great builder. Two projects which he initiated were completed in 1976, after he retired: a new pathology laboratory and radiation therapy facility, named for William A. Meissner and financed by a HEFA mortgage, and a new home for the School of Nursing, in honor of Audrey K. Kennedy, a long-time patient of Lyman Hoyt and then of Jim Tullis, and a Deaconess benefactor. Following Audrey Kennedy's death in 1968, a $500,000 bequest from her will initially made the new nursing school building possible. And thanks to the influence of Hoyt and Tullis, the Frederick J. Kennedy Foundation subsequently gave another $2.5 million while the hospital's trustees voted to transfer $937,000 of unrestricted funds. Colby Hewitt, a Deaconess trustee and excellent fund-raiser, then headed a campaign which quickly

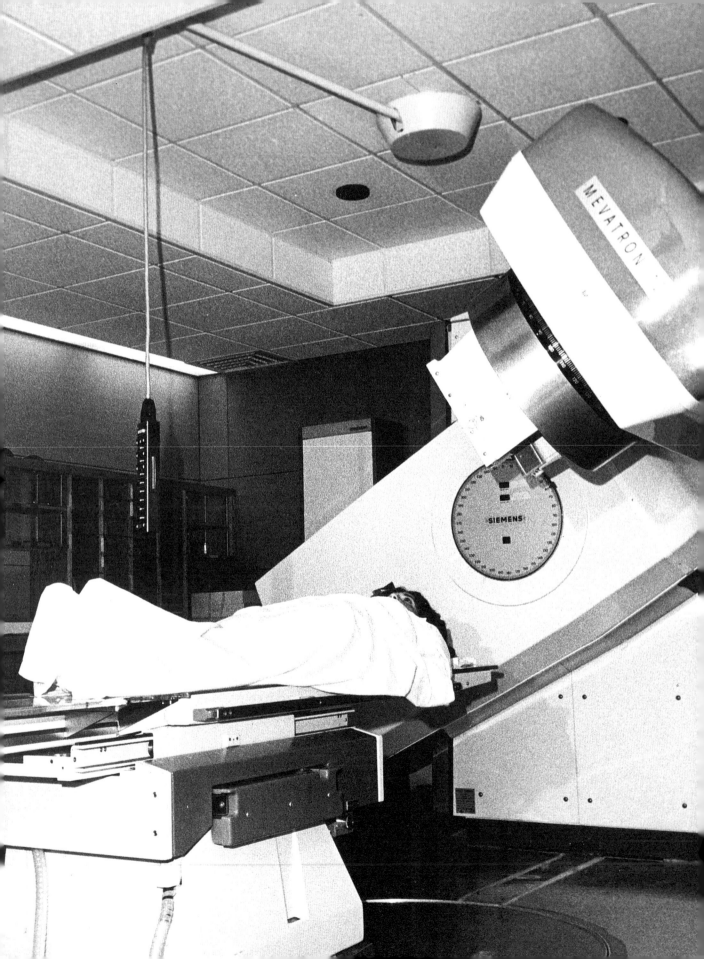

raised the remaining $1.3 million needed to complete the building, exceeding the hospital's goal by more than $200,000.

Both the Meissner and Kennedy buildings were state-of-the-art facilities. The Meissner Laboratory, which comfortably accommodated staffs for both clinical and anatomic pathology as well as the latest technology, arose on the site of Norwich House, which was torn down after psychiatry's relocation to the fourth floor of the Deaconess Building. The basement of the Meissner Building housed the Department of Radiation Therapy, which was part of the Joint Center for Radiation Therapy and had the latest equipment, including a 12MeV linear accelerator and other sophisticated technology.

Kennedy Hall, on Autumn Street, contained living accommodations for nurses as well as classrooms, a library, and an auditorium. At the dedication ceremony, the school's alumnae association surprised Ellen Howland by naming the auditorium in her honor. "We revel in the space, both inside and outside," Howland remarked, "and we delight in the ability to schedule classes, conferences, and meetings without using a slide rule. But we are most grateful for what the building represents, the visible affirmation of trustee and administration support for diploma education and for their faith in the quality of our school of nursing." Indeed, it was hard to question the school's excellence. In June 1975, its graduates scored first out of fifty-two diploma schools in Massachusetts on examinations in medicine and surgery given by the Board of Registration in Nursing.

Howland may well have had her fingers crossed when talking about the school's future, however, for she knew that the building had been purposely designed so that it could be converted to another use with relative ease. Although the trustees and administration had given a vote of confidence to diploma education, they had hedged their bets somewhat, realizing that baccalaureate curricula were growing in popularity and that the day might come when the hospital would no longer want to maintain a diploma program.

Don Lowry has recalled that one of the primary motivations behind his early retirement was his frustration over the red tape that the hospital had to cut through before it could proceed with the new buildings. State authorities had to issue certificates of need and the

THE 12MeV LINEAR ACCELERATOR *was one of the first high-energy machines used for treating patients in the Harvard Medical area. Considered one of the workhorses of the Joint Center for Radiation Therapy, it was employed for over a decade to treat thousands of people suffering deep-seated malignancies such as cancers of the lung, bowel, and prostate. Its electron capabilities were also suitable for use as superficial radiation, i.e., limited penetration of tissue in the treatment of skin cancer.*

projects had to win municipal approval as well. These processes consumed two years during a time of rapidly rising construction costs. The delays, Lowry estimated, added a million dollars to the cost of completing each project. Even a 345-space addition to the Pilgrim Road Garage had to receive a certificate of need before the hospital could build it in 1979. Since he had come from the regulated industries of banking and securities, MacLure found the regulatory process that was engulfing hospitals less aggravating than Lowry had; he was more used to rolling with the regulatory punches.

In 1976 the Joslin Diabetes Foundation, as the Joslin Clinic was now formally called, opened a new clinical wing, which it dedicated to Howard Root, Joslin's medical director from 1952 until his death in 1968. This addition was not funded by the Deaconess, but its completion allowed for an expansion of the Diabetes Treatment Unit (formerly the Hospital Teaching Unit), which was run and staffed by the Deaconess. The Joslin Clinic remained a major source of patients throughout these years, though the Joslin was also moving more heavily into research, where its ties were primarily to the Department of Medicine at Peter Bent Brigham Hospital. In 1977, Robert F. Bradley, Jr., the clinic's medical director since 1968, succeeded Alexander Marble as president. A new generation of leaders was in place.

Although the Deaconess took a breather from major construction projects after Kennedy Hall and the Meissner Laboratory were completed, it did have an ongoing renovation program. In 1978, for example, the hospital's maintenance and engineering department, with design recommendations from management and professional staff, built a new ambulatory care and observation unit on the first floor of the Deaconess Building. Two years later the Cardiac Catheterization Laboratory moved to larger, modernized quarters, while two operating rooms were renovated. Similarly, the hospital's lobby and entrance and some patient floors were improved, elevators were upgraded, a bridge connecting Harris Hall to the Farr Building was built, new treatment units were added, motel rooms in the Lowry Building were converted to doctors' offices, and a materials handling facility was opened in a former automobile dealership on Brookline Avenue behind Harris Hall.

In 1980 an 8,000-square-foot addition to the Cancer Research Institute was also erected, initially housing the laboratory of George H. A. Clowes, Jr., though additional space was reserved for use by a new chief of medicine. The CRI addition came under a newly enacted exemption to certificate-of-need legislation for research facilities and was financed primarily through special solicitations to individuals and foundations and secondarily through the sale of property the hospital owned.

MASSACHUSETTS WAS HARDLY ALONE in regulating new construction in these years. By 1972, twenty-three states had enacted certificate-of-need legislation. The American Hospital Association promoted such legislation as a way of encouraging greater planning and controlled competition among hospitals. By the mid-1970s, Massachusetts hospitals were required to file one- and five-year plans with the state. At the Deaconess, in 1975, Paul Babcock became the first staff planner.

In the absence of a strong political will to stop expansion, determination-of-need activities met with limited success in reducing duplication of facilities or services. Moreover, though politicians and regulators urged cost-containment upon hospitals, they also encouraged debt financing by allowing capital costs to be reimbursed through patient bills. Since third-party payors — usually government, private insurers, or Blue Cross — not patients themselves, actually paid the bills, there was little consumer pressure on the political system to rein in costs. On the contrary, the public wanted to maintain the hospital care to which it had grown accustomed and expected new lifesaving procedures and technologies to be readily available.

By 1980, the health-care industry accounted for 9 percent of the gross national product. "Despite the growth of bureaucratic controls, designed in many instances to contain health care costs, the costs of medical and hospital care have continued to increase at a rapid rate," Schorr and MacLure accurately reported in 1981.

The Deaconess was no exception and regulation did not impede growth of the hospital's budget. The Deaconess's operating revenues grew from $37 million in 1975 to $116 million in 1984, a threefold increase in ten years. Although the Deaconess experienced small operating losses a few times, it generally showed a year-end surplus: in 1983, $2.8 million; in 1984, $5 million. One constant, except for a slight dip during the year after the Lahey moved out, was that the Deaconess continued to operate essentially at capacity, with 93 or 94 percent occupancy and sometimes even higher, reportedly the highest rates in Boston.

AUDREY K. KENNEDY BUILDING, CA. 1980. Completed in 1976, Kennedy Hall succeeded Harris Hall as the new home for School of Nursing students.

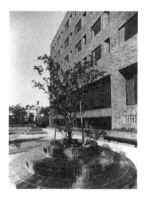

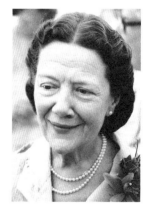

ELLEN D. HOWLAND at the dedication of the Audrey K. Kennedy Building, 1976. To honor the longtime Deaconess nursing leader, the alumnae association named the Kennedy auditorium in Howland's honor.

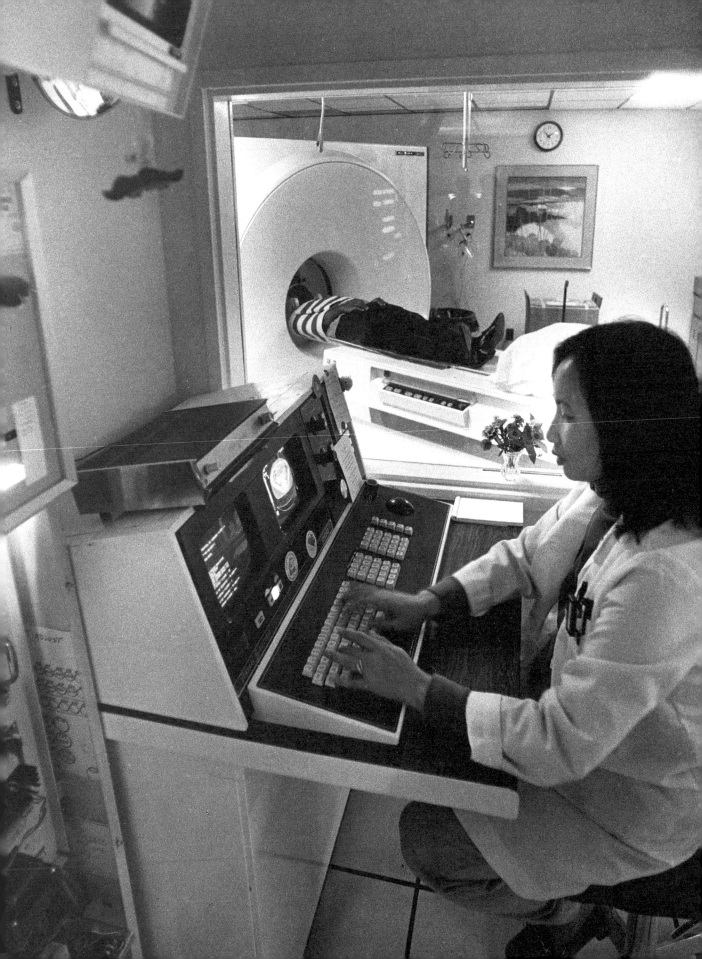

The regulatory thicket did, however, often slow the proliferation of technology at the hospital. Diagnostic radiology was a perfect case in point. The field of radiology was making dramatic progress, which the Deaconess was prepared to embrace as each new modality was proven effective. Between 1975 and mid-1979, the hospital spent $400,000 on nuclear medicine equipment and $150,000 on ultrasound technology, and was expecting an outlay close to $800,000 on a CT (computerized axial tomography) scanner, pending regulatory approval. The state's Public Health Council eventually authorized the purchase of CT scanners by only six area hospitals, including the Deaconess. Within a month of its installation in October 1980, the machine was scanning twelve patients a day — from the Deaconess, and from Mount Auburn, New England Baptist, and Brookline hospitals as well. The Deaconess's willingness to offer additional institutions access to the CT scanner was a factor in winning Public Health Council approval.

RECRUITING NEW CLINICAL LEADERS

With the arrival of the Harvard Surgical Service and the establishment of Deaconess Medicine, the hospital was able to strengthen its residency programs, recruit new staff, and move closer to Harvard Medical School. The appointments of young chairmen in medicine and surgery in the 1980s, both of whom came from major Harvard teaching hospitals, would not so much establish as affirm the course the hospital had embarked upon in 1973 and 1974. These young chairmen would probably not have considered coming to the Deaconess had the basis for a promising academic future not already been laid by the time the jobs became available.

Deaconess Medicine grew from a staff roster of four and a half physicians in 1975 to twelve two years later, though its growth rate then slowed pending the arrival of a new department chairman, after which it accelerated sharply. The surpluses generated by Deaconess Medicine allowed the hospital to recruit and support promising young subspecialists in several areas. In the fifteen years following Tullis's appointment as chairman in 1964, the number of medical residents increased from eighteen to fifty-two. For the purpose of education and

COMPUTERIZED AXIAL TOMOGRAPHY (CT) SCANNER, CA. 1980. *First introduced into service at the Deaconess in 1980, the CT installation was a joint project with other area institutions, including New England Baptist, Mount Auburn, and Brookline hospitals. Despite the scanner's slow scan time, the hospital eventually serviced between twenty-five and thirty patients a day on the GE 8000.*

coordination of patient service, the Deaconess Department of Medicine was organized into twelve sections: cardiology, pulmonary, renal, gastroenterology, neurology, hematology, oncology, endocrinology, rheumatology, allergy, psychiatry, and broad-based primary-care internal medicine. Implicit in this was the further expansion of subspecialization within American medicine.

Because the Deaconess was largely a tertiary-care, referral institution, not a general hospital, it was necessary to maintain affiliations with other institutions to round out the training of residents. With the arrival of the Harvard Surgical Service, four institutions affiliated immediately with the Deaconess: Cambridge, Mount Auburn, Faulkner, and the Manchester Veterans Administration hospitals. Cambridge and the Manchester VA were eventually utilized for training of Deaconess residents in medicine as well.

Some residents also went to Roxbury Dental and Medical Group one afternoon a week for a year to gain exposure to community health and primary care. The Roxbury Dental and Medical Group (RDMG), a community health organization, had been established in 1969 by two idealistic Deaconess doctors, surgeon Bradford Patterson and internist Donnell Boardman. The Deaconess provided the center with ongoing managerial and financial assistance. In 1972 a quarter of its operating budget came from the Deaconess; ten years later that proportion had grown to 30 percent.

A number of Deaconess physicians and surgeons practiced at the Roxbury center in the 1970s and 1980s, including Blake Cady, Laurence P. Cloud, T. Corwin Fleming, Randolph Reinhold, Arturo Rolla, and Clement Yahia. Much of their time was donated. Patterson and Boardman also provided service, but Patterson subsequently moved to Rochester, New York, where he became a professor of surgery, and Boardman concentrated on the Acton clinic where he was primarily affiliated. "RDMG was unique," said Reinhold, who served as its first executive director, "because it was one of the few centers in the country that tried, by choice, to provide quality medical care for low-income people in the city without federal funding, and with limited financing from private sources and the Deaconess." The involvement of the hospital and its staff members in this group demonstrated that the charitable impulse still breathed, the strong trend toward business values in health care and hospitals notwithstanding.

An outside review of the Deaconess's medical residency program highlighted the need to give residents greater exposure to psychiatry.

Consequently, in 1977, Miles Shore, a full professor at Harvard and chief of psychiatry at Massachusetts Mental Health Center, accepted responsibility for administering the section in psychiatry at the Deaconess. Paul Hans, a psychiatrist also based at Massachusetts Mental Health, moved his office to the Deaconess and developed a thriving practice. With their psychoanalytic and psychodynamic orientations, Shore and Hans broadened psychiatric practice and teaching at the Deaconess.

IN THE 1970s, the Department of Medicine also began to provide continuing medical education for senior physicians, which had been mandated by state law, and it became involved, though in a fairly limited way, in the training of Harvard medical students. The department still conducted only a modest amount of research, at least in comparison to full academic departments of medicine at Harvard. Nor was teaching fully incorporated into clinical activities, since there were many staff physicians who would have resisted such integration. Although Tullis himself had strong academic affiliations at Harvard Medical School, the department he headed did not have full status as an academic entity; probably only a minority of its members held clinical appointments at Harvard. Clinical appointments in medicine at the Deaconess still came through the chief of medicine at Peter Bent Brigham Hospital, Eugene Braunwald, who firmly believed that he should continue to do so.

The department's junior status at Harvard presented both a problem and an opportunity when the hospital began its search for a new chairman in 1978 — Jim Tullis hoped to retire in 1979. It made it harder to persuade top academicians to consider the job. But it also allowed MacLure to negotiate with Daniel C. Tosteson, the new dean of Harvard Medical School, over what would be required for the department to achieve full status at Harvard as well as a time frame for the decision. Tosteson agreed to set up a review procedure within five years of the appointment of a new chief, "with the expectation that the New England Deaconess Hospital will have a Harvard Medical School Department of Medicine at that time."

The search committee for the new chairman concluded that the hospital would be at a disadvantage in attracting the best candidate if hospital tenure were not included as part of the agreement. The hospital's trustees concurred. A few doctors were ardently opposed to the idea and they gathered enough signatures on a petition to call a special meeting of the medical staff in January 1979. At this assembly, however, a motion opposing the chairman's tenure was overwhelmingly rejected by those present. This vote represented an endorsement by the staff of the strategy that the hospital's lay and medical leaders had embarked upon seven years before. It also vindicated their gradualist approach to winning its acceptance.

In the spring of 1980, MacLure and Roger A. Perry, Jr., an associate director of the hospital with responsibility for fund-raising and external affairs, paid a visit to the Mallinckrodt Company and Foundation in St. Louis, a leader in the chemical industry. MacLure and Perry returned with a financial commitment toward the establishment of an endowed chair at Harvard Medical School in honor of Deaconess pathologist Shields Warren to be named the Shields Warren–Mallinckrodt Professorship. Warren agreed that the chair's first occupant would be the new chief of medicine at the Deaconess; thereafter, the holder would be a pathologist. As it happened, Warren died unexpectedly on July 1, 1980, at the age of eighty-two, having just completed another of his many scientific papers.

ALTHOUGH HE WAS A GRADUATE OF HARVARD MEDICAL SCHOOL and had spent most of his career at Massachusetts General Hospital, Robert C. Moellering, Jr., had never set foot in Deaconess Hospital before arriving to be interviewed for the chairmanship of medicine in 1980. In fact, that was the first time he even knew exactly where the Deaconess was — what he had learned from colleagues at Mass General was that the Deaconess was not an academic institution. A nationally prominent infectious disease specialist, Moellering, who was promoted to full professor of medicine at Harvard, was a member of the editorial board of the *New England Journal of Medicine* and the author of many scientific articles. He had turned down a chair at Johns Hopkins for personal, family reasons. While he was happy at Mass General and wanted to stay in Boston, he was in his early forties and interested in a new challenge.

Moellering was quickly impressed with MacLure and with what he was trying to accomplish at the Deaconess. Moellering was reassured by members of the Harvard search committee and by Dean Tosteson himself of their commitment to making the Deaconess an academic institution with full rank. Indeed, the Deaconess could not have gotten Moellering without

Tosteson's help. The search committee unanimously recommended Moellering and he was appointed Shields Warren-Mallinckrodt Professor of Clinical (later changed to *Medical*) Research. He was also granted tenure by the Deaconess, which meant that the academic portion of his salary was guaranteed by the hospital. MacLure promised him adequate research space, and Moellering subsequently moved his laboratory to the Cancer Research Institute. In addition, he was made head of Deaconess Medicine, which he was authorized to expand. Moellering came to the Deaconess full time in June 1981, succeeding Tullis, who had stayed two years beyond his desired retirement date.

Non-confrontational in style, Moellering was not interested in driving out or discouraging the hospital's private practitioners. His purpose was to build an academic department and he believed that private practice and full-time academic medicine could co-exist, which coincided perfectly with the hospital's long-range plan. One of the strongest divisions in medicine at the Deaconess, gastroenterology, headed by Charles Trey, preferred to remain private, as did the allergy division under Albert L. Sheffer, and a number of others. Moellering, however, had to ask several division chiefs to step down because their academic credentials were not strong enough.

Moellering recalled receiving immense help from several private practitioners who remained outside of Deaconess Medicine, including Ivy DeFriez, Arturo Rolla, and Burns Roehrig. Although Moellering had worried about his ability to attract top-flight academicians, recruitment proved easier than he expected. In 1982 he brought in two new division chiefs from Mass General, A. W. Karchmer in infectious disease, who began to recruit outstanding specialists and build a premier program, and Robert S. Lees in peripheral vascular disease. The following year, he recruited Jack W. Hawiger, an internationally known hematologist from Vanderbilt University, to run a research program in experimental medicine.

In addition, Moellering appointed Steven R. Goldring as section chief in rheumatology and hired Richard M. Rose as head of the pulmonary division, Ronald C. Silvestri as medical director of the intensive care unit, Joseph D. Zibrak as director of respiratory therapy, and Russell Vasile for inpatient psychiatry. Other recruits included

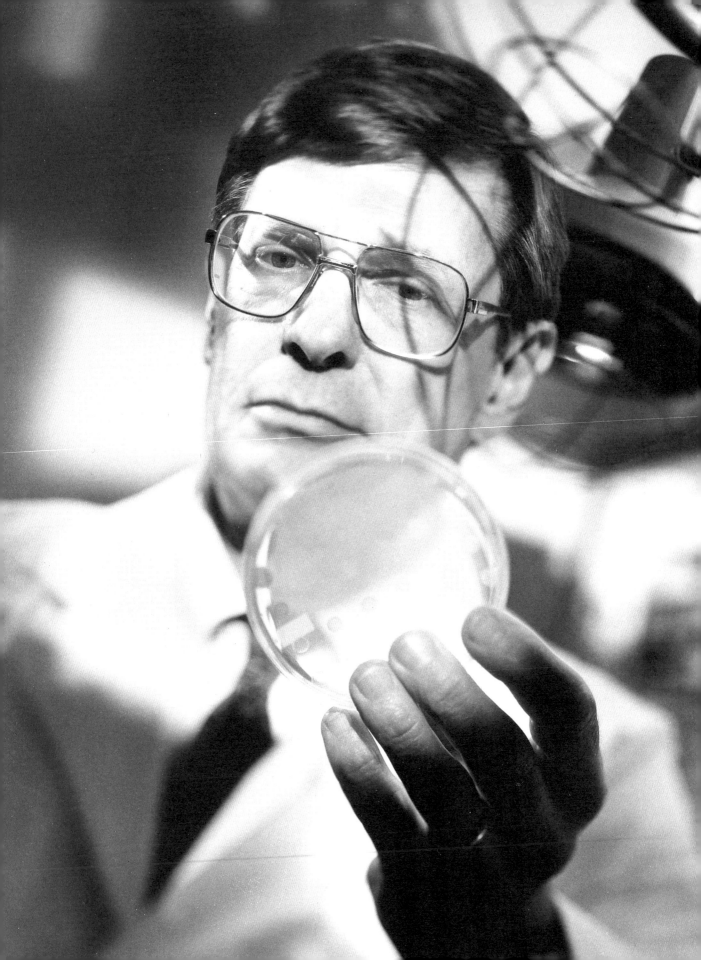

Z. Myron Falchuk, a nationally recognized gastroenterologist; the Blackwell Associates, an all-women's medical group, whose organizer, Judith Waligunda and two other members, Kim Bowman and Marian Klepser, were graduates of the Deaconess residency program in medicine; and oncologist/hematologist Jerome Groopman, whose important research on AIDS quickly attracted national attention and brought the hospital many patients suffering from this disease.

Each time Moellering was able to recruit a talented physician, it made it easier to attract the next one. In 1982, the research funding for the department was $800,000; two years later, it had grown to $4.7 million. In 1984, the department received more than a thousand applications from top medical schools for just thirty internship positions. In addition to more than forty second- and third-year residents, the department had over thirty specialized clinical and research fellowships. Under the direction of rheumatologist Lee S. Simon, and with assistance from the Department of Surgery, the Department of Medicine offered a revamped physical diagnosis course to second-year Harvard Medical students, who gave it the highest rating of any course at Harvard Medical School. Thus, Moellering soon lived up to expectations and moved quickly to establish a first-rate academic Department of Medicine deserving of full status at Harvard.

IN 1980 THE TRUSTEES GAVE BILL McDERMOTT a three-year term as chairman of the Department of Surgery, succeeding Neil Sedgwick, who subsequently moved out to Burlington with the Lahey Clinic. Tony Monaco followed McDermott as scientific director of the Cancer Research Institute. But McDermott was approaching retirement age; he was sixty-three at the time. The chairmanship was a way of acknowledging his large contributions to the hospital and it allowed for the unification of the clinical, teaching, administrative, and research functions in one person, thereby setting the stage for the appointment of a full-time, academic chief of surgery within a few years. By 1982, the department's very popular residency program was receiving 300 applications for 14 positions. Moreover, a number of the program's best graduates had decided to join the hospital's staff.

In 1982 Dean Tosteson appointed an ad hoc committee to recommend a successor to McDermott as professor of surgery and chief

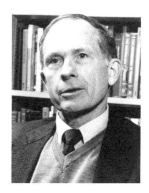

DR. DANIEL C. TOSTESON, CA. 1988. *Dean of Harvard Medical School since 1977, Tosteson has been an important supporter of the Deaconess and its role as a major teaching hospital of Harvard Medical School. Tosteson was instrumental in gaining full academic status for the Deaconess Department of Medicine.*

Facing page: Dr. ROBERT C. MOELLERING, JR., Chairman of the Deaconess Department of Medicine. A nationally prominent infectious disease specialist, Moellering succeeded James Tullis as chairman of medicine and head of Deaconess Medicine in 1981.

of the Department of Surgery at the Deaconess. The committee was chaired by Bob Moellering and included Carl Hoar, Laurie MacLure, Charles Schmidt, Marv Schorr, and Frank Wheelock from the Deaconess, and the chiefs of surgery from Mass General, Beth Israel, and Brigham and Women's Hospital, which had been created in 1980 out of a consolidation of the Peter Bent and Robert Breck Brigham hospitals and Boston Hospital for Women (Lying-In). Several other prominent Harvard Medical School professors served as well.

Before beginning its search, the committee surveyed the strengths and weaknesses of the Deaconess Department of Surgery. The major strengths it found were in the "superb caliber of the clinical care provided by an exceptional staff." Some committee members saw weaknesses in the residency program due to rotations to other hospitals, necessitated by the highly specialized nature of the Deaconess, but on the whole felt that the program worked well and attracted outstanding candidates. The department's major shortcoming was seen as the lack of a mechanism for generating funds to support programs in clinical care, teaching, and research. Without such a modus operandi, the committee felt that the department would be in a poor position to get a worthy candidate to head it and assume a professorship. Consequently, despite the misgivings and doubts of some of the hospital's private surgeons, the Deaconess Board of Trustees approved in principle the establishment of a hospital-based group practice in surgery, comparable to what it already had in medicine.

The committee conducted a wide-ranging search, inviting six candidates for visits and interviews, four of whom were asked back for additional meetings. At the conclusion, in the summer of 1984, the committee selected Glenn D. Steele, Jr., an associate professor at Harvard and a surgical oncologist at Brigham and Women's Hospital who was also affiliated with the important new Dana-Farber Cancer Institute. A Harvard graduate, Steele had gone to New York University School of Medicine and had served his internship and residency at the University of Colorado Medical Center. Under a special NIH Fellowship, he had taken two and a half years off from his residency

to do research under Hans Sjorgen in Sweden and earned a Ph.D.
in immunology from Lund University.

Steele was only forty years old in 1984, but he had already
done significant cancer research, was a popular and effective teacher, and
had developed a substantial referral practice. Because he was a busy
clinician as well as an active researcher, Steele later sardonically observed,
he did not fit the stereotype of the "academic rat doctor." Although he
was younger than the other finalists, his youth was seen as an asset
because it was felt that he would be motivated to build the department
and that he would be able to attract other top young surgeons.

Prior to his appointment at the Deaconess, Steele had been on
the verge of moving to Columbus, Ohio, where he was to head a new
cancer hospital at Ohio State University. He had, however, indicated that
he would accept the Deaconess offer if it came before he moved, which
it did by a mere two weeks. For Steele, the Deaconess presented a perfect
opportunity, allowing him to maintain his scientific collaborators and
clinical referral sources, while opening wider research possibilities. The
Deaconess already had an excellent reputation in secondary and tertiary
care, which is what Steele was himself doing. Given the age structure of
the department, he also felt he could build a strong academic program
without having to displace people. In January 1985, Steele became chairman of surgery while assuming a new professorship at Harvard named for
William V. McDermott, which had been established with funds provided
by McDermott's many friends, patients, colleagues, and former residents.

BY THE TIME OF STEELE'S APPOINTMENT, a number of other departments
had undergone leadership changes as well. In 1975 Melvin E. Clouse
had been made chairman of diagnostic radiology, succeeding Mirle A.
Kellett who, after twenty-seven years at the Deaconess, had decided
to move to Maine, where he spent summers. A tall, good-humored
Texan, Clouse had been an X-ray technician before going to college
and medical school. Following a residency and fellowship at Mass
General, he came to the Deaconess in 1969 to perform vascular and
interventional radiology.

Six radiologists comprised the department when Clouse became
its chairman; they drew about three-quarters of their income from the

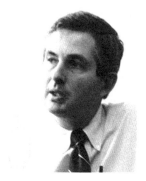

*Dr. Glenn D. Steele, Jr.,
ca. 1985. Assuming the
chairmanship of the Department of Surgery in January
1985, Steele was named the
William V. McDermott
Professor of Surgery at Harvard
Medical School. Steele's skills
as a clinician, researcher, and
teacher were all highly valued
by the hospital. His administrative leadership brought new
vigor to the department,
consolidating clinical strengths
and expanding research and
teaching efforts.*

hospital and about one-quarter from the private practice group to which they belonged. By 1984, this group had been folded into the hospital and all department members were full-time members of the hospital staff. Important technological breakthroughs were already reshaping the field of diagnostic radiology; the department housed subspecialties in mammography, nuclear medicine, angiography, and ultrasound.

Clouse supported the direction the hospital was taking, in part because diagnostic radiology itself was becoming a more exciting academic field. He chaired the Medical Administrative Board from 1979 to 1981, from which he helped quash the last flurry of opposition to the hospital's new role when tenure was being granted to the new chairman of medicine. Clouse had also reinstated a small residency program and the department offered fellowships in several subspecialties.

From a modest beginning, the department's training programs, headed by Herbert F. Gramm, soon flourished. Within a few years, they had achieved national recognition and were inundated with highly qualified applicants. By 1984, radiology had nine residents and five fellows. Clouse stimulated and encouraged his colleagues to conduct research and publish papers, and he and his colleagues, including Gramm, Philip A. Costello, Robert A. Kane, and Daniel H. O'Leary, worked closely with surgeons to devise new techniques and procedures. A group of what had been primarily clinical radiologists gradually developed into academicians.

Unlike radiology, the Deaconess Department of Radiation Therapy, which was affiliated with the Joint Center for Radiation Therapy, had a significant academic orientation from the beginning. From an original group of about ten, by 1983 the Joint Center had grown to 130 full-time employees, seeing 3,000 new patients annually from the Longwood area hospitals as well as from the Faulkner Hospital in Jamaica Plain. The Deaconess typically supplied the most patients, although others were not far behind: more patients were treated at the Deaconess than anywhere else — 43 percent — in 1980. By 1983, more than sixty physicians had been trained as radiation therapists, three of whom had already become department chairs at prominent medical schools. With fourteen residents each year, the Joint Center for Radiation Therapy had become one of the premier training programs in the country.

Since 1968 both Deaconess radiation therapy and the Joint Center had been chaired by Samuel Hellman. Given Hellman's remarkable record of accomplishment and his widespread recognition, it is not surprising that other institutions became interested in hiring him. In 1983, Hellman resigned from the Joint Center and the Deaconess to become physician-in-chief at Memorial Hospital, Sloan-Kettering Cancer Center in New York City, the nation's leading cancer research hospital. Subsequently, he was named dean of the University of Chicago Medical School. After Hellman's resignation in 1983, Jay R. Harris became acting chairman while Harvard Medical School launched a search for Hellman's successor.

Research conducted by the Joint Center led to new treatment programs for Hodgkin's disease and to the introduction of lumpectomy/radiotherapy treatment for breast cancer. In collaboration with MIT, the Joint Center also pioneered in dynamic treatment — computer-controlled radiotherapy — which maximizes the dose to a tumor while minimizing the effect on healthy tissue. (In close cooperation with the Deaconess Department of Surgery, in 1981 the Joint Center pioneered in the development of intraoperative radiation therapy, creating the country's first such unit.)

The Department of Pathology had a long history of academic leadership under both Shields Warren and Bill Meissner. Bill Meissner retired as chairman in 1972, but remained active as a clinician, teacher, and researcher. The chairmanship then rotated between Bradley Copeland and Merle Legg until Copeland left Boston for personal reasons in 1979. Under Copeland and Legg, the department continued to have a large residency program and to perform a high volume of clinical work for the Deaconess and other hospitals. Members of pathology did important research work in these years in a number of areas, including the definition of certain tumors. In 1980, pathology generated $13,500,000 in revenues. The department also consulted widely — over 2,000 times in 1980 — and it set high standards for quality, winning national and international recognition in the process. That year Legg directed the annual Anatomic Pathology Seminar in St. Louis, the country's largest pathology program.

In contrast to other areas, anesthesiology had remained divided at the Deaconess between a private practice group, Anaesthesia Associates of Boston (under Leo Hand and Francis Audin), and the

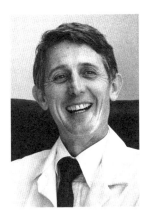

DR. MELVIN E. CLOUSE, CA. 1977. *Succeeding Mirle A. Kellett as chairman of radiology in 1975, Clouse was named a full professor at Harvard Medical School in 1988. Today the Deaconess Department of Radiological Sciences is a leader in the use of state-of-the-art radiological technologies. Clouse's own work includes contributions to interventional and vascular radiology.*

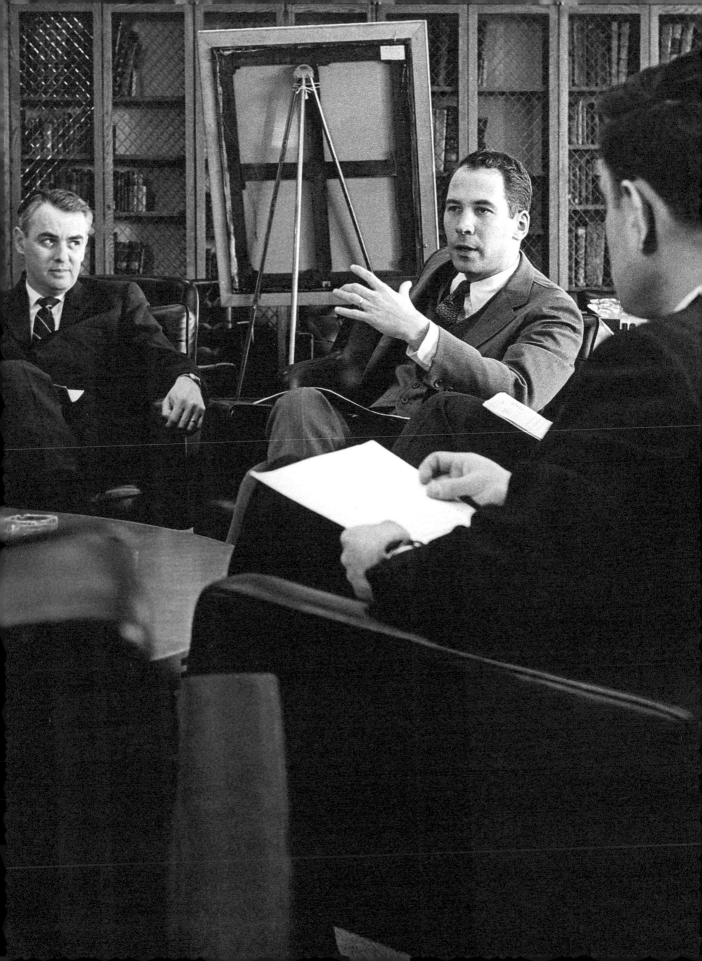

anesthesiology department of the Lahey Clinic. Both groups performed excellent clinical work, and each had its own residency program. By the early 1970s, the Lahey Clinic had trained about 160 residents and Hand/Audin about 60; but both training programs were subsequently closed. Their termination was part of a movement promoted by the American Board of Anesthesiology toward medical-school-based residencies. Nationally, the number of anesthesiology residency programs shrank by more than 40 percent in these years.

The closing of the residency programs led to the utilization of anesthesia care teams. In this system, certified registered nurse anesthetists (CRNAs) essentially replaced residents. The CRNAs, like the residents who preceded them, worked under the continuous medical supervision of anesthesiologists. When the Fifth Harvard Surgical Service moved to the Deaconess, staff anesthesiologists began to provide instruction to all surgical residents. Eventually Harvard voted to establish a Department of Anaesthesia separate from the Department of Surgery, of which anesthesiology had always been a part. Harvard's affiliated hospitals followed suit, including the Deaconess, which in 1982 named a renowned patient safety leader, Ellison C. Pierce, Jr., as chairman. The new Department of Anaesthesia (and its professional practice group, Anaesthesia Associates) provided all anesthesiology services for the Deaconess. The group was also asked to take over services at the Faulkner Hospital and expanded significantly to meet the growing demand.

The Department of Surgery meanwhile continued to oversee the Division of Podiatry, which was headed in the 1970s and 1980s by Rob Roy McGregor, John C. Donovan, and Geoffrey M. Habershaw, successively. McGregor initiated a residency program at the Deaconess in 1972, with rotations to many other Boston-area hospitals. The program achieved national recognition and its graduates found themselves in considerable demand. While vascular surgeons were achieving remarkable results for diabetic patients, podiatrists also continued to contribute a great deal to foot care for diabetic and non-diabetic patients alike.

DR. SAMUEL HELLMAN (center), new head of the Joint Center for Radiation Therapy, confers with members of the press and directors of the four founding hospitals, including Beth Israel, Boston Hospital for Women, Peter Bent Brigham, and the Deaconess, 1968. At left is Richard Lee, director of Deaconess Hospital.

END OF AN ERA: THE LAHEY CLINIC DEPARTS

"On November 24, 1980, Lahey Clinic Medical Center opened its own 200-bed hospital in Burlington and, as a result, reduced its daily bed utilization at our hospital from approximately 135 to about 25," Schorr and MacLure wrote in the 1981 Deaconess report. "Fortunately, we had ample notice of this rather dramatic shift in demand and the obvious implications for our traditionally high occupancy levels." MacLure reported to the Board of Trustees that hospital occupancy for the nine months following Lahey's departure was 80 percent. Despite the drop in occupancy, however, the hospital still managed to exceed its demand forecast and showed a $2.3 million surplus for the year. The Deaconess took advantage of the Lahey's departure to renovate patient and operating rooms.

Although the hospital's management was able to report a positive result at year's end, the Lahey Clinic's departure did produce tense moments along the way. "I really thought that the bottom might fall out of this hospital on December 1 when their last patient left," MacLure later acknowledged. In the year preceding its move to Burlington, Lahey management had steadily lowered its estimate on the number of beds it would need at the Deaconess, raising anxiety levels within Deaconess management correspondingly. Moreover, while the Deaconess had in a sense been preparing for the Lahey's departure ever since the creation of the Long-Range Planning Committee and the adoption of the Tullis plan, there was no way of knowing for certain how things would turn out once the Lahey actually left.

The Lahey Clinic continued to utilize the Deaconess on a limited basis for both medical and surgical patients after it moved to its new medical center. This was dictated in part by the fact that the clinic had not yet received certification from the state for cardiothoracic surgery or kidney transplants in Burlington and in part to a shortage of beds for internal medicine and psychiatry in its new location. Lahey neurosurgeons also continued to perform some operations at the hospital. The clinic was responsible for 49,250 patient days at the Deaconess in 1980, 15,225 in 1981, and 5,755 in 1982. Although the pull-out was not total, the trend-line was dramatically downward.

The departure of the Lahey Clinic left a great many empty beds, which were largely filled by the general surgical and medical staffs, including Joslin and Overholt Clinic members. A number of doctors who had previously hospitalized some of their patients elsewhere, sometimes because beds at the Deaconess were hard to come by, now gladly admitted them. By September 1981, MacLure reported to the Board of Trustees that the hospital had, remarkably enough, achieved a 94.9 percent occupancy, based on the 472 beds that were then open. "The beds are filled as follows: Lahey 18, Joslin 129, Overholt 18, general staff 275 and residents 8." In January 1981, Deaconess Medicine was filling 60 beds a day.

Arriving full time seven months after the Lahey moved out, Bob Moellering conducted a rigorous hiring campaign. In 1982, thirty-three physicians joined the Department of Medicine, twelve as members of the associate staff. Before that surge in hiring, the Deaconess had been modestly augmenting its staff in anticipation of the Lahey's move. Mel Clouse told the corporation's annual meeting in January 1981 that the Lahey's departure presented short-term problems, while also opening up long-term opportunities for the hospital to develop its medical staff and add new subspecialties.

When the Lahey Clinic left, not every one of its staff members wanted to go; several chose to enter private practice and thereby remained affiliated with the Deaconess. A few approached hospital management with the idea of becoming full-time employees of the hospital. Only one, Blake Cady, a highly regarded cancer surgeon, was hired in this capacity, however. Cady went to Burlington initially, but wanted to return to the Deaconess to teach and do research; he did not want to be restricted to clinical work, which remaining at the Lahey would have meant. He later rose to the rank of full professor at Harvard Medical School. Cady's hiring encountered some resistance from surgeons who feared it was the opening wedge for a full-time academic department, which in a way it was. MacLure and McDermott put it through, however, without undue strain.

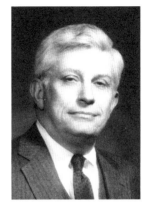

DR. ELLISON C. PIERCE, JR., CA. 1990. *A national leader in patient safety, Pierce became chairman of the Department of Anaesthesia in 1982. Pierce served as president of the American Society of Anesthesiologists and the Anesthesia Patient Safety Foundation, and was honored for his work by the Surgeon General of the United States in 1989.*

A NEW AND COMPETITIVE ENVIRONMENT

In the late 1970s and early 1980s, there was a realization within the Deaconess, as elsewhere, that a new competitive environment was ahead for hospitals and health-care providers. When Ronald Reagan was inaugurated President in 1981, MacLure remarked to the annual meeting of the Deaconess corporation on the new administration's commitment to reducing taxes and rolling back regulation. "If planners and politicians shift from regulation as the answer to cost containment, to competition between hospitals and other types of providers, hospitals may lose the protective benefit of regulation while at the same time gaining a certain amount of freedom in the forms of competition and risk."

In the late 1970s, Jim Tullis and hospital officials had begun to think about how referral patterns might change. The impressive growth of health maintenance organizations, especially in Massachusetts where Harvard Community Health Plan was establishing itself as a leader, and the increasing importance of subspecialization and technology, which not all hospitals could afford, both suggested that more referrals would be institution-to-institution rather than doctor-to-doctor. This was especially true of a specialty-referral hospital, such as the Deaconess, which drew its patients from a wide geographic area.

Thus the Deaconess began to establish relationships with outlying hospitals, including St. Luke's in New Bedford, Massachusetts, and Portsmouth, Wentworth-Douglass, and Frisbie Memorial hospitals in New Hampshire. The Deaconess supplied these institutions with services they lacked, such as oncology and hematology, and they, in turn, referred complicated cases to the Deaconess. In addition, the Deaconess developed a relationship with Brookline Hospital, a nearby community hospital which was struggling to survive, a struggle it would ultimately lose. Deaconess staff members had also conducted continuing education programs at Monadnock Community Hospital in Peterborough, New Hampshire, for more than twenty years, and that association helped generate referrals. In addition to fostering good institutional relationships, Tullis, Sedgwick, and others believed that it remained important to have an active staff on the cutting-edge of medicine, publishing papers and giving lectures.

The new competitive environment also suggested that hospitals might have to merge and consolidate in order to weather growing external pressures. Multi-hospital systems and hospital chains were on the rise nationally, among both non-profits and for-profits. In step with this trend, the Deaconess initiated merger talks with New England Baptist in 1979, but the Baptist, which had maintained a more traditional approach, decided to remain independent. The Deaconess also began to explore ways of delivering services other than at the hospital itself, such as through ambulatory surgi-centers and home health care services. But complex and highly specialized surgical and medical procedures continued to be central to the Deaconess's mission and distinctiveness.

Ushering in a new era

Exciting developments in organ transplantation in the early 1980s helped solidify the Deaconess's position as a first-rate tertiary-care, referral hospital. In 1970 Tony Monaco had performed the hospital's first kidney transplant, and by the early 1980s, the Deaconess had become one of the principal kidney transplant centers in New England, performing about sixty transplants annually, many in collaboration with the Joslin Diabetes Center. During these years, a number of Deaconess internists and surgeons closely followed attempts elsewhere to transplant livers, and several Deaconess doctors collaborated in experimental transplants on animals. Liver transplants were extremely difficult procedures, however, with high rates of rejection and failure. Francis D. Moore, chief of surgery at Peter Bent Brigham Hospital, had attempted several but abandoned them as unfeasible. In 1979, however, the introduction of a new anti-rejection drug, Cyclosporin A, began to improve survival rates for human patients. In 1982, the one-year survival rate at the University Health Center in Pittsburgh, the largest liver transplantation center in the world, was 70 percent.

The dramatic improvement in results led to the establishment of appropriate committees at the Deaconess to formulate plans for the

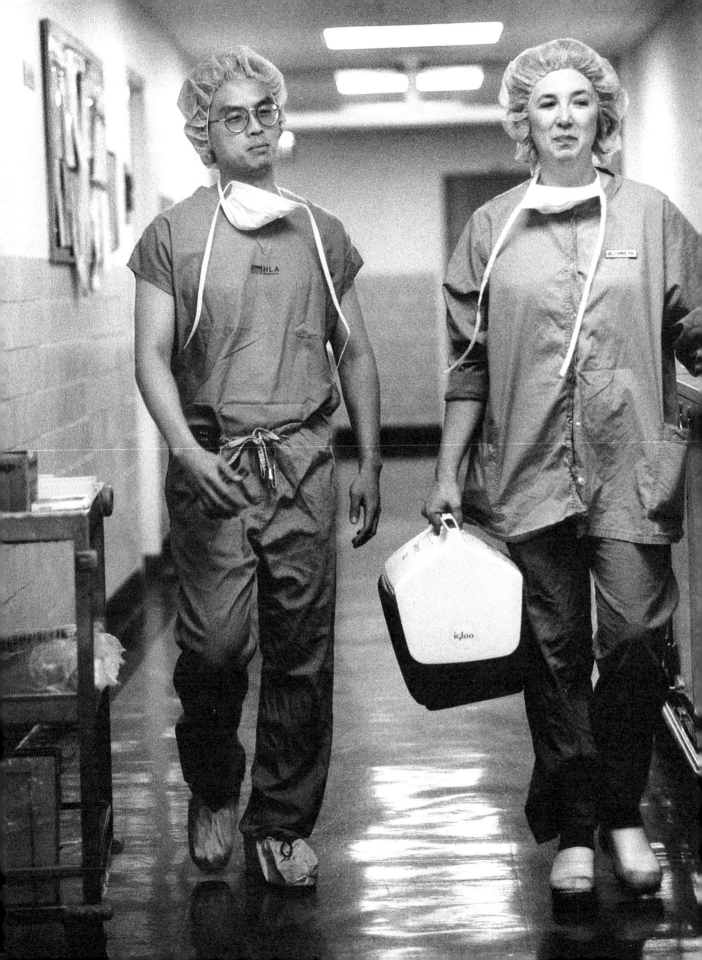

initiation of its own liver transplant program. At MacLure's behest, planner Paul Babcock prepared a lengthy and careful business plan for such an endeavor. Although the hospital had a wealth of experience in renal transplants and in liver surgery, Bill McDermott, who specialized in liver disease, insisted that the Deaconess not attempt a liver transplant without adequate preparation and training. He respected the difficulty of the procedure, the most rigorous and demanding of all transplants, and believed it would be unethical to experiment on patients. Moreover, failure could hurt the hospital's reputation in the medical community.

As a result, McDermott asked Roger Jenkins, who had just completed the hospital's residency program and was regarded as extraordinarily able, to go to Pittsburgh to train under Thomas E. Starzl, head of the liver transplant program there. Jenkins had been planning to do a fellowship in cardiothoracic surgery, but was attracted by the challenge of becoming the liver transplant team leader at the Deaconess. He spent five months working closely with Starzl, gaining invaluable experience in harvesting as well as transplanting livers. In addition, the Deaconess sent other doctors, nurses, and technicians to Pittsburgh for shorter durations to learn about the particular problems involved in this procedure. The hospital carefully trained and readied its team.

There was no shortage of people who desperately needed liver transplants; gastroenterologist Charles Trey, widely respected in his specialty, had a number of patients who suffered from primary biliary cirrhosis for whom a transplant was the only hope of survival. Regulatory and financial impediments initially barred the door, however. The Massachusetts Department of Public Health appeared reluctant to authorize any hospital to perform the procedure on a regular basis. Massachusetts Blue Cross/Blue Shield meanwhile had classified liver transplants as experimental and would not cover surgical costs, which averaged between $70,000 and $100,000.

In the summer of 1983, the Deaconess petitioned the Department of Public Health for a waiver, allowing a liver transplant on Richard Pillin, a victim of primary biliary cirrhosis. Trey's patient since 1971, Pillin had been hospitalized many times over the preceding six months and entered the Deaconess in a coma on July 3. His liver

Members of the Hospital liver transplant team, Dr. Paul Kuo, fellow, and Jil Ferris, O.R. nurse, 1991. Since performing New England's first liver transplant in 1983, Roger Jenkins and the Deaconess team of surgeons, nurses, infectious disease specialists, social workers, and psychologists have led the region in liver transplantation surgery. Important research and clinical trials involving the Deaconess led to the approval of new drugs to improve survival rates for liver transplant recipients.

was ceasing to function; dangerous levels of nitrogen had built up in his blood. The state granted the waiver on the basis of the life-threatening situation. With the assistance of the Deaconess social service department, Pillin's brother successfully petitioned the state welfare commissioner for Medicaid funds to help pay for the transplant.

On the evening of July 13, Thomas Starzl and his colleague, Byers Shaw, in a magnanimous gesture, flew in from Pittsburgh at Jenkins's request to lend moral support and technical assistance. That night a harvesting team of Starzl, Blake Cady, and Peter Benotti rushed to Lawrence General Hospital to procure a liver from an accident victim. As soon as that team confirmed that the organ was suitable, a surgical team at the Deaconess led by Roger Jenkins and including Albert Bothe, Tony Monaco, and Ira Fox, along with Pittsburgh's Byers Shaw, began to remove Pillin's diseased liver. The harvesting team arrived at 4:00 A.M. with the donor organ in excellent condition and by 8:30 A.M., Jenkins and his team had implanted it.

News of the operation gripped the hospital's medical and nursing staffs throughout that night and the following day. In the afternoon, McDermott, Jenkins, and Monaco met with the news media and announced that the Deaconess had successfully completed its first liver transplant. The story generated wide publicity, as did Pillin's discharge from the hospital at the end of August. Before Pillin left, Jenkins had performed a transplant on another patient, Edythe Trautz, this time without Starzl and Shaw present.

Meanwhile, McDermott had taken a lead role in organizing the Boston Center for Liver Transplantation, a cooperative effort of four hospitals — Children's, Massachusetts General, New England Medical Center, and the Deaconess. The center won a determination of need from the state, which allowed these institutions to perform transplants on a regular, rather than emergency, basis. During the first year of the center's existence in 1984, twenty-eight liver transplants were performed, almost half of which, thirteen, were at the Deaconess.

The liver transplant program reinforced the Deaconess's identity as a tertiary-care, referral, and academic institution. Indeed, the program grew directly out of the hospital's overall strategy. A carefully thought-out and executed plan allowed the Deaconess to position itself as one of the few hospitals in New England capable of doing these operations *and* permitted to do them.

The manner in which the Deaconess entered the liver transplantation field reflected institutional traditions of effective management and of the melding of excellent science with outstanding patient care. It manifested as well the increasingly challenging and competitive environment in which hospitals had to function.

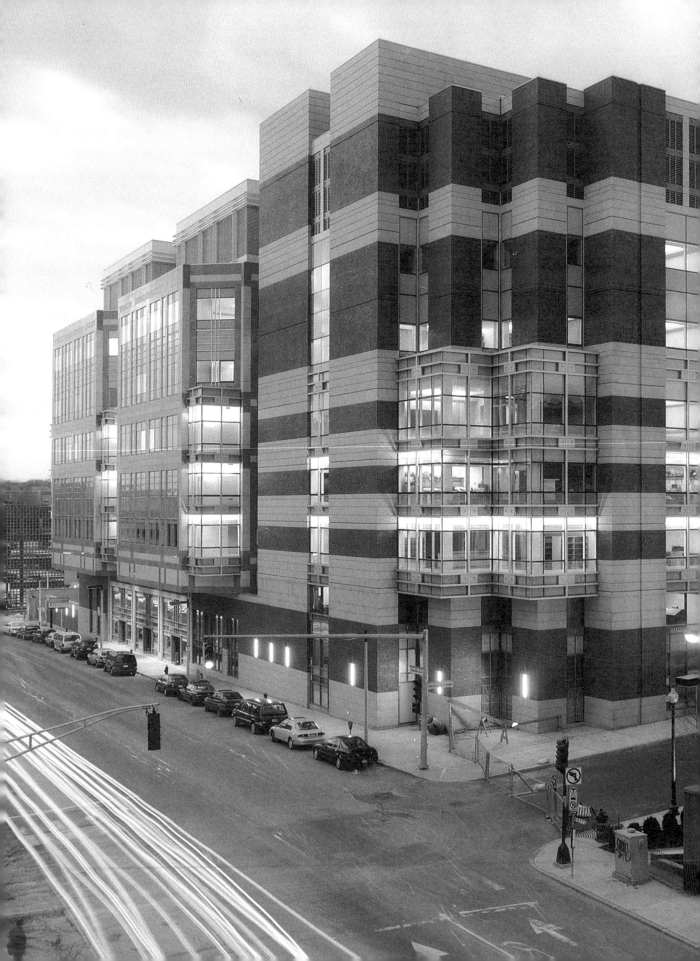

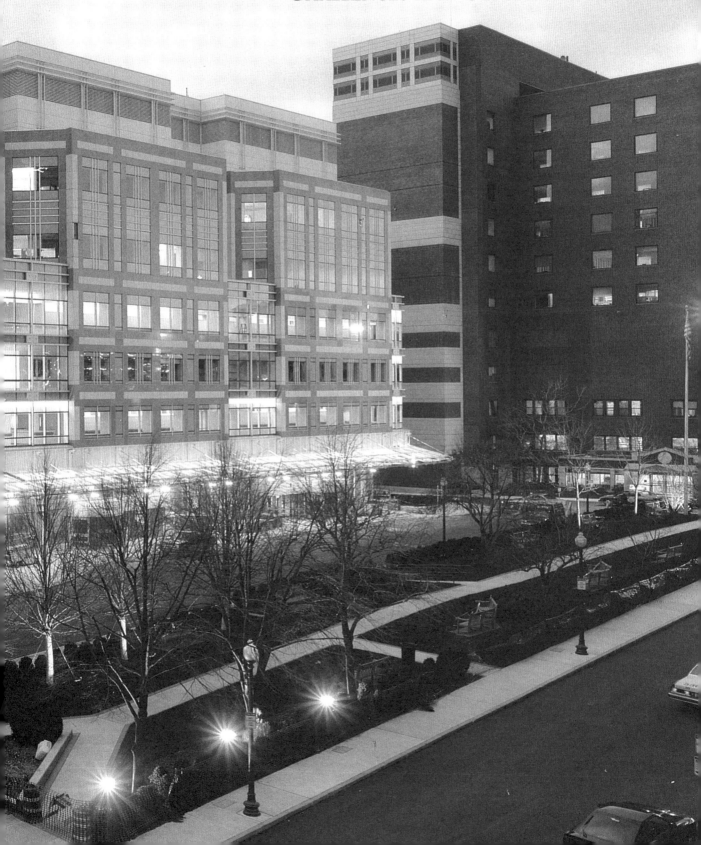

Overleaf:

Deaconess Hospital Clinical Center, 1994. Opened in January of 1995, the new Clinical Center was built to carry the Deaconess tradition of care well into the twenty-first century. With 330,000 square feet of space, the Clinical Center houses state-of-the-art facilities and sophisticated equipment and serves as the technological hub for Deaconess Hospital and Pathway Health Network. Designed by Shepley Bulfinch Richardson and Abbott of Boston, the structure resulted from seven years of careful planning, design, and construction.

CHAPTER FIVE:
CHALLENGES AND OPPORTUNITIES

By the late 1980s and early 1990s, the Deaconess had gained recognition as a top-quality academic and tertiary-care hospital with a distinguished medical staff. The long-awaited state-of-the-art Clinical Center was completed while plans for the development of a consolidated research facility were progressing. The Deaconess was poised to enter its second century supported by both the wisdom of experience and the vision of new leadership. But this period of maturation and development was also marked by enormous challenges as fundamental changes in health care were beginning to emerge.

A DIFFICULT DECISION

By 1985 the presence of energetic young heads of medicine and surgery, Robert Moellering and Glenn Steele, respectively, each with mandates to increase their staffs and expand research activities, virtually required that the Deaconess examine how well its physical plant was meeting both current and future needs. The hospital had growing numbers of clinicians and researchers who were practicing on site as members of the staff or one of its professional practice plans. The Lowry Medical Office Building had been adequate when many attending physicians still had their offices elsewhere; now the facility lacked the capacity to house the hospital's growing professional ranks.

The expansion of staff became necessary as admissions and occupancy began to decline slightly in the mid-1980s and new capabilities were added to keep pace with expanding and changing needs. The slippage in admissions had several sources: the retirements of several senior clinicians; the growth of health maintenance organizations and changes in reimbursement methods, which discouraged admissions and urged shortened lengths of stay; and the increasing competition for patients among Massachusetts hospitals. Inpatient utilization in the Commonwealth declined by 27 percent between 1983 and 1991. If the Deaconess wanted to generate the funds necessary to support physical revitalization of the hospital plant, it would need to find effective ways to manage within the new health-care climate and the growing emphasis on efficient utilization of beds and services.

The Deaconess leadership recognized that the hospital's physical plant no longer met the needs of modern medicine. Operating rooms built in the

the 1950s were too small to accommodate comfortably either the technology or the number of people needed to perform the sophisticated procedures of the 1980s and '90s and beyond. The hospital's intensive care units were likewise in need of updating. Facilities for diagnostic radiology, where technology continued to burgeon, were inadequate and inefficiently located. Outpatient facilities were also wanting as it became both possible and desirable to provide sophisticated services, such as cardiac catheterizations and chemotherapy, on an outpatient basis. While research grants were expanding significantly, research space was static. Laboratory and office areas had to be leased off campus, which did not promote cohesiveness or strengthen the ties between research and clinical care.

With assistance from consultants Marvin Bostin and the architectural firm of Payette Associates, the Long-Range Planning Committee presented a master facilities plan to the trustees in early 1986. The study called for the erection of a new patient-care building where Harris Hall stood and recommended the development of expanded outpatient facilities, space for additional medical staff offices, and increased research areas. In looking at the overall feasibility of the plan, Bostin and Payette Associates also raised the question of whether the School of Nursing was the best use for Kennedy Hall.

As a result of the consultants' recommendations, the trustees authorized then board chairman Colby Hewitt to appoint an ad hoc committee of trustees, management, and other appropriate individuals to study the future of the Deaconess School of Nursing and utilization of Kennedy Hall. Board member John P. Hamill was named chairman of the committee, which included Laurens MacLure; trustees Helen Chin Schlichte, John I. Carlson, Jr., Marvin Schorr, and Colby Hewitt; Merle Legg, chairman of the pathology department; Barbara Hooker, the nursing school's recently appointed director; Elizabeth Zappelli, a member of the school's faculty; and Marion Metcalf, a Deaconess alumna and director of nursing at Peter Bent Brigham Hospital. Joyce Tower, assistant director of the hospital for operations, served as staff.

The committee's deliberations took place against the backdrop of a twenty-year national debate over the future of nursing education, a debate which had divided nurses and their member organizations. The American Nurses' Association, a national organization, advocated making the baccalaureate degree a prerequisite for "professional nursing" and the associate degree the prerequisite for "technical nursing," and proposed eliminating diploma and practical nurse programs altogether. In contrast, the National League for Nursing, the accrediting agency for all nursing education programs, supported multiple-entry routes to nursing. In 1983 a congressionally mandated two-year study by the Institute of Medicine advocated educational mobility and opposed artificial barriers to academic upgrading.

In the face of the increasing popularity of baccalaureate programs, however, Hamill and other members of the committee were concerned about the long-term outlook for the School of Nursing. Although the quality of students had remained high, by 1986 total enrollment had dropped to 140. There was no question that students were receiving a superb nursing education at the Deaconess. Indeed, over four consecutive years 100 percent of the school's graduating classes had passed the licensure examination and scored very well on national tests.

Although the hospital subsidized the school financially, relative to the Deaconess's total budget the support was small. There was concern, however, that federal financing of nursing education might soon be reduced or eliminated, which would increase the hospital's burden. Hiring Deaconess graduates saved the hospital in recruitment and orientation efforts. Of these new hires, however, only about a quarter remained at the Deaconess for more than five years. At the end of 1985, a little more than a third of the Deaconess's 508 registered nurses, including 24 members of the school's faculty and staff, were graduates of the school. Although the school's presence eased recruitment for the Deaconess, other Boston hospitals which had closed their diploma schools had managed to remain fully staffed.

Some committee members took an interest in preserving the school by moving it off campus or by merging it into a college or university, but neither idea appealed to Barbara Hooker and other advocates for the school. They cherished the wonderful facility they had in Kennedy Hall as well as the school's reputation and tradition. Merging the school would have effectively ended it as a distinct institution and as a diploma program, which had been the fate of a number of other diploma schools. Hooker felt the committee should make a clear-cut decision — either keep the school or close it. She also did not want to

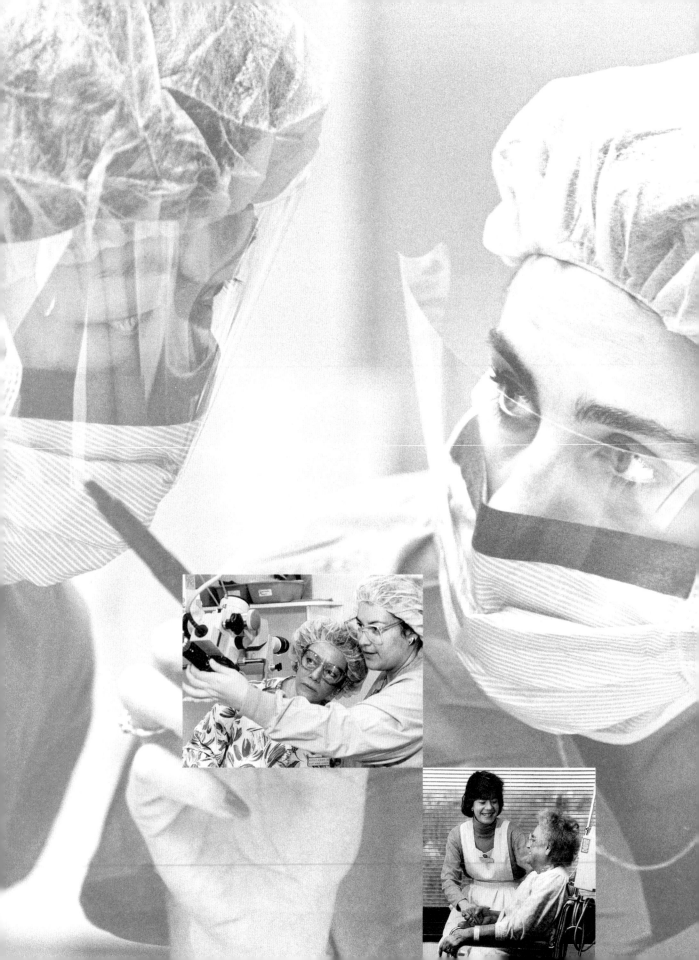

delay judgment, for if the school were to be retained, student recruitment would have to begin at once.

In the end, the committee reached a consensus to close the school. They did so advisedly and with regret, but in view of trends in nursing education and, in light of the hospital's pressing space needs, closing made sense. "Obviously, in the best of all worlds, the School would remain and contribute in the future as it has so marvelously in the past," anaesthesia head Ellison Pierce wrote Department of Pathology chairman Merle Legg. "However, one must weigh all of [the School's] significant advantages against the very strong need of adequate facilities for the current and future programs in the clinical departments. Both Dr. Moellering and Dr. Steele are presently building very strong staffs in many, many areas. They clearly are limited in this task by the inadequate physical facilities at the hospital."

Laurens MacLure recalls, "The decision to close the School of Nursing was one of the most difficult in the history of the hospital." Indeed, the nursing school had been an integral part of the hospital since the beginning; the Deaconess Home and Training School, its forerunner, had, of course, preceded establishment of the hospital itself, so closing the school was bound to be an anguishing decision. Among alumnae, there was understandable sadness and even anger at the outcome. Ellen Howland and Barbara Hooker were realists, however, loyal to the hospital, and stateswomen as well. "This is a very difficult time for everyone associated with the school," said Howland, who had been the school's director for twenty-nine years. "We knew that hospital schools had been closing across the country for many years, but we hoped that ours would continue as long as we could attract qualified students and faculty, which we have continued to do."

Rather than being shut down overnight, the school was phased out in an orderly and thoughtful manner. The last class entered in the fall of 1986, as planned, and graduated three years later, in May 1989. Thanks to a generous incentive severance plan, the faculty remained on board and accreditation was maintained throughout.

IN LATE 1985, SIX MONTHS BEFORE THE DECISION to close the nursing school, Judith Miller was hired as associate director of the hospital and

MODERN NURSING practice at the Deaconess continues to find ways to redefine the role of nurses in the delivery of health care. In addition to planning and managing patient care, Deaconess nurses are involved in every facet of clinical activity. Research in nursing practice has resulted in changes in hospital policy and patient-care delivery.

chief nursing officer. Miller had worked at the Deaconess for six years in the 1970s, instructing first-year nursing students while she herself pursued a master's degree at Boston University. She then rose to nursing care coordinator and nursing supervisor. Miller subsequently moved to Texas where she held hospital administrative positions. Miller recognized that it would be a "no-win" situation for her to become enmeshed in the controversy so soon after she arrived. She therefore asked not to be appointed to the committee, believing that she would be in a stronger position to deal with whatever the outcome if she had not become identified with one position or another.

Miller's hiring coincided with the start of a new era in nursing care. While nurses have remained actively involved in direct patient care, increasingly they have also filled the vital role of patient-care managers, planning and coordinating care for a group or a floor of patients. Patient-care technicians and other support personnel have assumed many of the non-clinical tasks previously performed by nurses. Yet despite the sea changes in the profession, nursing has retained its traditionally strong role within the Deaconess. Today, nurses furnish a myriad of services and assume increasing responsibility central to the provision of patient care. Thus it is not surprising that on a larger organizational scale, Miller eventually assumed responsibility for all Deaconess patient-care services, not just nursing. The changes in nursing care have not affected patients' attitudes about the Deaconess. According to recent surveys of patient satisfaction conducted by the hospital, the tradition of compassionate care established by the original deaconess caregivers is alive and well. More than 96 percent of patients responding to surveys have given especially high marks to Deaconess nursing. Overall, Deaconess care has substantially exceeded the norm for teaching hospitals nationwide.

A FINANCIAL SETBACK

Just a year after making the decision to close the nursing school, the Deaconess encountered disturbing and unexpected financial problems precipitated by the fact that Massachusetts, which had previously enjoyed an exemption, entered into the Medicare Prospective Payment System. Under the federal system, hospitals were reimbursed for Medicare patients according to Diagnostic Related Groups (DRGs). The reimbursement formulas were complex and hospitals were subject to audit for several years after their performance of services, at which time they might be found to have overcharged. It therefore became necessary for hospitals to reserve funds for such contingencies. The question of how much to put aside, however, was not clear.

The hospital's 1987 budget was based on reimbursement assumptions which by the spring, six months into the fiscal year, were beginning to prove much too optimistic. Admissions were down, case intensities and length of stay were up, and so therefore were expenses. The Deaconess had the highest proportion of Medicare patients — nearly half its patient population — of any of the major teaching hospitals in Boston.

When it became clear that revenue projections were not being met, MacLure and Lee asked the hospital's outside auditors to assess the situation. As a result of their preliminary findings, MacLure informed the trustees in May that on a year-to-date basis the hospital had lost $3.2 million, whereas it had expected to show a gain of $2.8 million. He anticipated a year-end loss of $6 million, though he also indicated that it could be double that amount.

The financial setback came as both surprising and disturbing news to the trustees. During the previous twenty years, there had been losses in only four, with a combined total of a little over $1 million. The bad news took the trustees' breath away, MacLure recalled. Although he subsequently offered to resign, the unexpected financial difficulty actually ended up postponing his retirement by two years. In 1986 MacLure had informed the trustees' executive committee that he hoped to retire in July 1987, when he would turn sixty-two. MacLure and the trustees concurred that the financial situation needed to be reversed first or the hospital would be in a poor position to conduct a search for his successor. It was decided that MacLure himself was the best person to rectify the situation. The trustees' budget committee, chaired by John Hamill, met frequently with MacLure and other senior managers, and became closely involved in designing the hospital's turnaround.

MacLure and the trustees recognized the signs that fundamental changes had to be made. Once they realized that the hospital was going to incur a loss in 1987, they decided, with the participation and approval of the hospital's outside auditors, to recognize a number of third-party

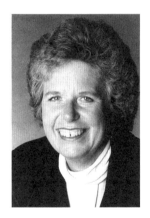

JUDITH R. MILLER, CA. 1991.
As senior vice president for patient-care services, Miller has influenced the evolving role of nurses and other hospital caregivers. A national leader in nursing, Miller served as president of the American Organization of Nursing Executives and in 1995 was named a fellow of the American Academy of Nursing.

issues which represented liabilities generated from the current or prior year's operation, so that the hospital would never again be negatively influenced by retrospective third-party reimbursement audits. In effect, the trustees chose to get all the bad news behind them. They switched from a very optimistic course to a conservative policy of acknowledging and booking third-party liabilities.

In the wake of the financial woes, the hospital's management instituted a number of cost-cutting measures to reduce expenses and minimize layoffs. An early retirement program was offered and more than 100 long-time employees participated. Although this added more than $6 million to the hospital's 1987 deficit, it was a one-time cost and reduced expenses subsequently. A hiring freeze was implemented, certain clinical services were pared back or reorganized, purchases and salary increases were delayed, and several benefits were reduced. Task forces were established to work on improving productivity and increasing patient volume. All of these efforts required cooperation among management, doctors, and nurses. In addition, in 1988 William J. Robinson was hired as the new chief financial officer, becoming a key member of the hospital's senior management and reporting directly to the president.

The following fiscal year, 1988, proved harrowing. Although people inside the Deaconess had been informed by the fall of 1987 of the hospital's financial problems, word spread widely after publication of the annual report in January. Key staff members heard from growing numbers of institutions interested in hiring them. J. Robert Buchanan, general director of Massachusetts General Hospital, approached the Deaconess board about a possible takeover, while Harvard Community Health Plan made overtures toward establishing a major relationship. The Deaconess rejected both suitors.

Nineteen eighty-eight had begun with great uncertainty because of the expiration of both the state's laws governing reimbursement and the master Blue Cross contract, which was closely tied to these regulations. But new health-care legislation allowed reasonable increases in reimbursement and the Massachusetts Rate Setting Commission approved a favorable retroactive rate adjustment. In addition, the hospital's internal task forces produced favorable results. Admissions rose 7.1 percent over the previous year while the average length of stay dropped from 10.7 days to 9.5. Surgical procedures and outpatient visits both increased. Various cost-saving measures also helped.

For MacLure, the most worrisome aspect of the crisis was not correcting the hospital's finances — he was confident that could be accomplished — but whether there would be an exodus of key professional staff, especially the chiefs and their excellent new recruits. If that were to happen, the hospital could find itself in a serious downward spiral. Fortunately, the chiefs remained on board, testimony in no small measure to their confidence in MacLure and the hospital. Indeed, instead of dividing staff members, the crisis actually became a call for united action.

There were disappointments, to be sure. Most significant, the financial loss caused a postponement in the planned clinical care facility. The renovation of Kennedy Hall, a more modest project, did proceed close to schedule, however, and was rededicated as the Audrey K. Kennedy Ambulatory Care Center in 1990. At $7 million, the cost of converting this building to an outpatient facility turned out to be more than four times what the consultants had estimated in 1985. But there was no doubt that the space was well utilized by, among others, a new cardiology program, the divisions of General Internal Medicine and Infectious Disease, a clinic for HIV-related diseases, and the offices of a Blue Cross-sponsored HMO. In addition, the Gilbert Horrax Library moved into expanded space that the nursing school library had occupied.

A UNIFYING VISION

By August 1988, after it was clear that the hospital's finances were on the mend, a search for MacLure's successor could be initiated without the burden of an unsure financial outlook. John Hamill chaired the search committee, which included clinical chairmen Moellering and Steele; trustees James F. Morgan, Helen Chin Schlichte, and R. Gregg Stone; corporation member Kenneth S. Safe, Jr.; and Colby Hewitt, the chairman of the board, an *ex-officio* member. Roger Perry, a senior vice president who was expecting to retire soon himself, served as staff.

The committee hired a Chicago-based recruiter who specialized in matching top-level managers with hospitals. Hamill stressed that the search should be wide open, and although a doctor might be preferable, a medical degree was not a requirement; the committee was primarily interested in someone with leadership experience in a teaching hospital.

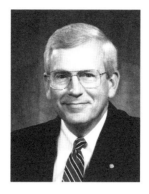

DR. J. RICHARD GAINTNER, 1990. *As the hospital's first physician-president, Gaintner brought a long career in academic medicine to his position at the Deaconess. From 1989 to 1994 he guided the hospital during a time of staff development, physical expansion, and financial and strategic challenges. In 1994 Gaintner became president and chief executive officer of Pathway Health Network, a new alliance of community-based physicians, hospitals, and health centers that he was instrumental in creating.*

By the following March, the committee had conducted a number of interviews and narrowed the search down to two finalists. But neither worked out as hoped and the search was resumed. The headhunter soon reported back on J. Richard (Dick) Gaintner, who had not previously been interested in the position. Circumstances were different, however, and Gaintner decided that he was ready for a change. Since 1983, he had been president and chief executive officer of Albany Medical Center, a 674-bed teaching hospital and free-standing medical school (Albany Medical College) that he was credited with developing into a regional tertiary-care and educational facility.

A graduate of Lehigh University and the Johns Hopkins School of Medicine, Gaintner had completed his internship and residency at University Hospital in Cleveland and a fellowship in hematology at Johns Hopkins. He had spent the major part of his career in administration, however, working in senior positions at Johns Hopkins Hospital and the Johns Hopkins School of Medicine and at New Britain General Hospital and the University of Connecticut School of Medicine before going to Albany. Over the years, he had also continued to teach.

When Gaintner came to the Deaconess for his first interview, he recalls, it was "almost love at first sight." He was as impressed with the members of the search committee as they were with him. Gaintner was quickly invited back for a second interview and then for a third at the end of June, when he was offered the job. Accepting immediately, he simply shook hands with John Hamill on the terms that had been discussed. Gaintner agreed to serve at the pleasure of the board, with no employment contract. The ease and informality of the negotiations boded well for the future: Gaintner's appointment became effective at the end of July 1989.

Several things had struck Gaintner about the Deaconess. Although many academic medical centers excel in the science of medicine, commitment to sensitive patient care is often absent. That was obviously not the case at the Deaconess, where both science and patient care mattered equally. Gaintner was impressed with the chiefs and with the high quality of the hospital's residency and research programs. He was also pleased with the way the hospital's management, board, and staff had dealt with adversities — the Lahey Clinic's departure, the decision to strengthen ties to Harvard, and the financial setback of 1987. Instead of wringing hands, people had pulled together to find solutions.

The search committee favored Gaintner because of his strong background in academic settings, the homework he had obviously done on the Deaconess, his past success at fund raising and institution building, and the strength of his personality. Although a medical degree had never been considered a prerequisite for the position, there was some feeling that it was important to place the Deaconess president on a par with the heads of most Harvard-affiliated hospitals. Members of the search committee and others were reassured by Gaintner's consensual style and by his understanding that physicians were critical to the hospital's organization and had to be involved in decision making.

Gaintner began at once to set his own agenda. Dick Lee, who had been chief operating officer for twenty-two years, had decided to retire from the Deaconess and subsequently became chief executive officer of a health-care group-purchasing organization. To succeed Lee, Gaintner selected Albert B. Washko, who had spent most of his career with the Veterans Administration, running the VA hospital in Albany and then, at a young age, advancing as a VA regional director, responsible for twenty-three medical centers in seven states and Puerto Rico. Washko was named executive vice president and ran the hospital day to day, while Gaintner concentrated on strategy, fund raising, and external relationships; he also worked directly with the medical staff. In addition, Gaintner brought Ralph Horky with him from Albany as senior vice president for planning and marketing and to serve as informal chief-of-staff.

Gaintner's first experiences at the Deaconess confirmed his initial impressions. The hospital's strategy, programs, operations, and finances were all in good shape. He was concerned, however, that the Deaconess lacked a clear, unifying vision and sought a way to put in words the hospital's longtime ethos. Gaintner understood the importance of articulating the hospital's values and value system clearly and cogently.

Gaintner discovered a fitting phrase while reading a 1940 history of the Deaconess published by the School of Nursing Alumnae Association. According to that chronicle, Mary Lunn and a committee from the Board of Managers of the New England Deaconess Home and Training School had been formed in 1894 "to plan a hospital where science and Christian kindliness should unite in combating disease." In 1989 the Deaconess staff and patients included a significant number of

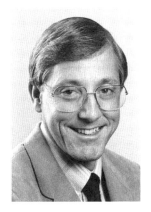

ALBERT B. WASHKO, 1990.
As executive vice president, chief operating officer, and later president, Washko has utilized a wealth of organizational skills in managing the operations of Deaconess Hospital. His long career in health-care administration proved critical in shepherding a major restructuring of hospital operations to assure quality while reducing costs in an increasingly competitive health-care environment.

individuals who were non-religious or who practiced religions other than Christianity. Gaintner recommended and the board agreed to omit the word "Christian." The modified quotation, which was attributed to Mary Lunn herself, assumed a prominent place in Gaintner's speeches, in the hospital's public relations efforts, and in its formal mission statement: "a place . . . where science and kindliness unite in combating disease."

A FOUR-PART MISSION

By the early 1990s, the Deaconess had succeeded in retaining key personnel and in attracting both accomplished physicians and promising young clinicians and researchers. The four sides of the hospital's expanded mission — teaching, research, clinical care, and community service — were flourishing, enhancing its reputation nationally and internationally.

During this time the Deaconess relationship with Harvard Medical School matured and deepened. Key appointments in medicine and surgery strengthened the academic focus. With both pathology and surgery as Harvard-affiliated departments, each establishing their own teaching, training, and research programs, the stage was set for more. In 1986 Harvard granted the Deaconess Department of Medicine full appointing status. This distinction did not happen quite as quickly as Bob Moellering had hoped or expected when he became department chairman five years earlier. Some of the chiefs at other major teaching hospitals had been reluctant to bring another to the table. Nevertheless, Harvard Medical School Dean Daniel Tosteson adroitly placed them on the committee to evaluate the Deaconess department, for he was confident that they could only come to a favorable conclusion; and they did.

In pathology, the historical ties between the medical school and the Deaconess continued with the 1988 appointment of Harvard professor Harvey Goldman to succeed Merle Legg as chairman. A serious illness had forced Legg to consider retirement. (Fortunately, he later recovered and was able to resume part-time work, which he continues to this day. In 1989 Legg and his wife, Dr. Yangja Jung-Legg, were instrumental in establishing an exchange program between the Deaconess and Xi'An University in China, an enriching relationship for both institutions.) When Legg's retirement was imminent, Laurie MacLure informed Dean Tosteson of the hospital's need to have a replacement without undue delay and suggested that it might make sense to appoint someone who was already a full professor at Harvard. A search committee subsequently selected Harvey Goldman, who had spent his career at Beth Israel. "It's an honor knowing my name will be in the company of such illustrious people as Shields Warren, William Meissner, and Merle Legg," Goldman remarked upon coming to the Deaconess in early 1989.

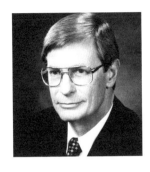

DR. ROBERT C. MOELLERING, JR., 1994. *In addition to overseeing the Department of Medicine, Moellering has continued important research on bacteria, gaining international recognition for his accomplishments. The recipient of numerous awards in his field, Moellering was elected president of the Infectious Diseases Society of America in 1991.*

TO CARRY ON THE DEACONESS TRADITION of providing excellent clinical care within an academic teaching center, over the last decade the hospital's department chairs have organized staffs of both outstanding clinicians and superb scientific investigators. Under Glenn Steele's leadership, the Department of Surgery has shown great vitality and strength. When Steele became chairman in 1985, the department was composed of outstanding junior and senior clinicians and researchers. As some of the more senior clinicians retired, Steele recruited replacements whose backgrounds in academic surgery would fit well at the Deaconess. From the beginning, Steele did not attempt to build a service that offered universal surgical care; rather, he concentrated on specialties where the department was already strong or could excel in the future. In the cancer field, for example, with important contributions by the chief of the Section of Colorectal Surgery Ronald Bleday, the Deaconess has made significant advances in clinical and research studies of solid tumors, colorectal and upper gastrointestinal cancers, and inflammatory bowel disease. Moreover, in seeking staff physicians, the department made a conscious decision to pursue qualified female candidates. The hospital took advantage of the increasing numbers of women surgeons and residents in training; in 1992, 32 percent of the Deaconess's surgical residents were women.

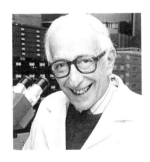

DR. HARVEY GOLDMAN, 1991. *A superb researcher and teacher, Goldman was named chairman of the Department of Pathology in 1989. As faculty dean for medical education at Harvard Medical School, Goldman was a principal architect of the New Pathway program, which prepares medical students to apply the expansion of scientific knowledge and technology to the practice of medicine.*

As department head, Steele decentralized decision making, shared administrative leadership, and created a system for rewarding institutional service as well as clinical activity. Inevitably there were some areas where things did not succeed the way Steele had hoped, such as the cardiothoracic division, where unifying private practitioners at the Overholt Clinic with full-time cardiothoracic surgeons proved an elusive goal. Overall, however, Steele and the department have built a strong and cohesive surgical service.

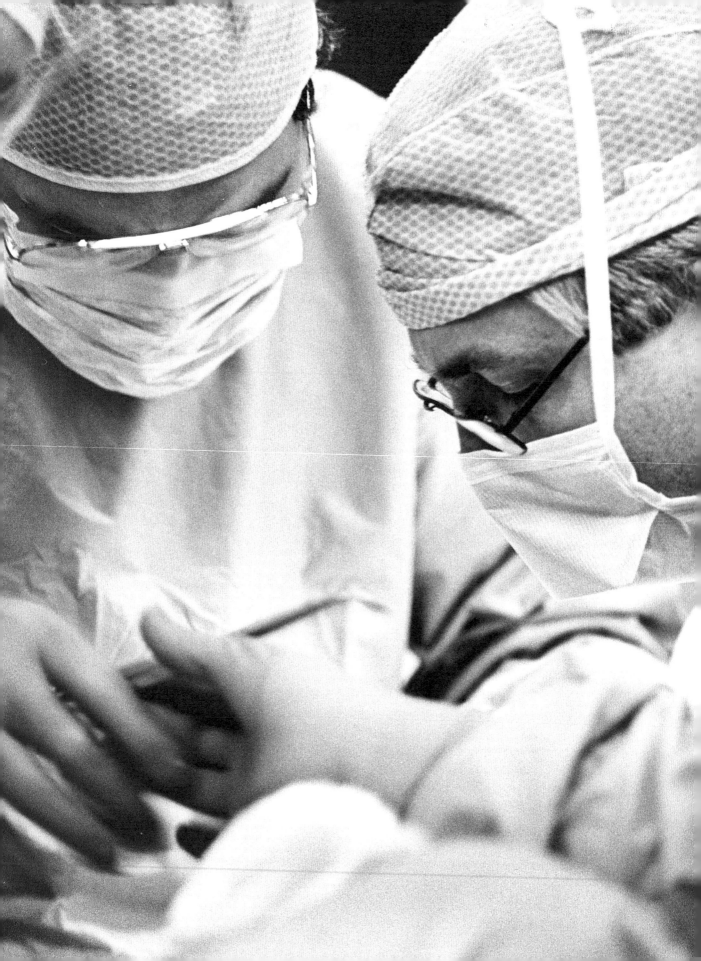

The current staff of Deaconess surgeons have helped pioneer and introduce a number of new techniques to reduce the trauma of surgery. Cardiothoracic chief and David W. and David Cheever Professor of Surgery Sidney Levitsky, for example, has developed techniques for myocardial preservation during surgery, with a special focus on the needs of the elderly patient. R. Armour Forse, the chief of general surgery, was an early leader in developing the new technique of laparoscopic surgery for excision of the gallbladder, placing the hospital in the forefront of the field.

Robert Eyre, chief of the Division of Urology, is a leader in urologic oncology, reconstructive urinary tract surgery, and male infertility and treatment of male sexual dysfunction. The division's recently established Laboratory for Reproductive Biology is involved in a number of projects, including research on HIV in the reproductive tract and the roles of prostate specific antigen and seminal vesicle specific antigen in semen.

Under Frank LoGerfo, the Division of Vascular Surgery, in collaboration with Joslin Diabetes Center, has become an international leader in the area of vascular reconstruction for patients with diabetes and related foot problems. Through the division's clinical and research efforts, the hospital's vascular team has achieved a 90 percent success rate with bypass grafts, dramatically reducing the incidence of amputations.

In the last several years the Deaconess has become the most active member of the Boston Center for Liver Transplantation. When Roger Jenkins performed New England's first successful liver transplant in 1983, he expected to do three to ten procedures a year. Seven years later it was not uncommon for Jenkins to perform two liver transplants *a week*. In the spring of 1990, Jenkins and the Deaconess team completed their 200th procedure, a milestone marked by few other hospitals; by early 1995, the total passed 350. With this vast clinical experience, researchers in hepatobiliary surgery are also working to maximize the effectiveness of liver transplants. Multi-institutional clinical trials involving the Deaconess led to the approval of a new immunosuppressant drug known as FK506 for all liver transplant recipients.

Maintaining quality of care while maximizing efficiency continues to be one of the main goals of the Department of Surgery.

DR. GLENN D. STEELE, JR., 1994 *(right)*. A renowned researcher and teacher as well as clinician, Steele has focused his own clinical practice on surgical oncology with a special interest in colorectal and gastrointestinal tumors. Steele's current research work in colorectal cancer and surgical oncology have received significant funding support. In 1993, Steele was elected to the Institute of Medicine of the National Academy of Sciences.

Ongoing quality assurance efforts, spearheaded by vascular surgeon Gary Gibbons, have led to the creation of Integrated Clinical Pathways (ICPs), a system for planning, delivering, monitoring, documenting, and reviewing patient care. Thus far, the ICP program has helped in controlling utilization associated with diagnostic and treatment procedures, providing consistency of care, and identifying patterns and trends based on variances from the norm.

In the Department of Medicine, infectious disease specialist and division chief A. W. Karchmer developed his division into a first-rate clinical service. In 1992 Karchmer was named a full professor at Harvard. Similarly, under Stanley Lewis, the clinical cardiology division has become a regional leader in interventional procedures such as cardiac catheterization, angioplasty, and coronary artery stents, among others.

Important research and clinical work have characterized the career of Bruce Bistrian, the chief of the Division of Clinical Nutrition. The department's seventh full professor, Bistrian is a past president of the Society of Parenteral and Enteral Nutrition, serves on various editorial boards in his specialty, and continues to make important contributions to the field.

In 1990 the Deaconess, in collaboration with Joslin Diabetes Center, named a new head of nephrology. As chief, Patricio Silva has recruited a strong team of clinicians and researchers while continuing his own work on renal handling of electrolytes. Endocrinology is another important area that exemplifies the long association between the hospital and Joslin Diabetes Center. The clinic's medical director, Gordon Weir, simultaneously served the Deaconess as chief of endocrinology into the early 1990s when he was succeeded by Edward S. Horton, who also followed Weir as Joslin's medical director. (Another sign of the closeness between the two institutions is demonstrated by the fact that Gaintner and Dr. Kenneth E. Quickel, Joslin's current president, serve on the board of each other's institution.)

The Department of Anaesthesia continues to be a national leader in the field of patient safety under the direction of Ellison Pierce, and since 1995 under Pierce's successor, Robert H. Bode, Jr. The Deaconess anesthesia team has earned a reputation for providing services of the highest caliber and has expanded their services to area hospitals. Deaconess anesthesiologists also play a central role in one of the hospital's multidisciplinary clinical programs. Along with staff from neurosurgery, behavioral medicine, and nursing, Deaconess anesthesia personnel form the core of specialists who treat patients with recurring pain at the hospital's Arnold Pain Center. Founded in the mid-1980s, today the center treats more than 500 patients annually for pain of all types — from chronic pain syndrome to cancer, neuropathic, and postoperative pain.

In the 1990s significant changes occurred in the practice of psychiatry at the Deaconess. Historically a division of the Department of Medicine, psychiatry became a separate department in 1991, joining medicine and surgery as an admitting service. Psychiatry's new status resulted in part from the creation of a consolidated department of psychiatry at Harvard Medical School under a new chairman, Joseph Coyle, recruited from Johns Hopkins. The departmental structure embraces several institutions, including McLean, Massachusetts Mental Health Center, Brigham and Women's Hospital, as well as the Deaconess.

Under a new department chief, Andrew W. Brotman, Deaconess psychiatry contributes its expertise and resources to the consortium in areas that are consonant with the hospital's mission, such as inpatient services, geriatrics, mood disorders, patients with medical problems who also require psychiatric care, and seriously mentally ill patients from the community. The Department of Psychiatry also serves an important role in the development of the new Harvard Longwood Residency Training Program by providing the primary site for training residents in inpatient psychiatric treatment.

SINCE THE MID-1980s, research support at the Deaconess has grown exponentially. In 1982, the Department of Medicine had research grants totaling $282,000. By 1986 that number had grown eightfold to $2.2 million and nine years later research funding had increased more than sixfold, to $13.8 million, about half of the hospital's research monies. Similarly, the Department of Surgery's thriving research program totaled $8.3 million in 1995.

The federal government, through the National Institutes of Health (NIH), has been and continues to be a mainstay for supporting hospital research programs. But cutbacks have occurred throughout government and the NIH budget, while it has increased, has not kept up with inflation and is today under serious threat. Despite this, Deaconess programs have continued to receive support: the Deaconess is now the

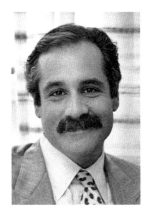

DR. ANDREW W. BROTMAN, 1992. *Named chief of the hospital's reorganized Department of Psychiatry in 1991, Brotman has overseen a major restructuring of services. Among the significant changes are the doubling of inpatient volume, expanded research collaborations, establishment of a residency training program, and a new emphasis on outpatient services to meet the growing needs of the revolution in managed-care services.*

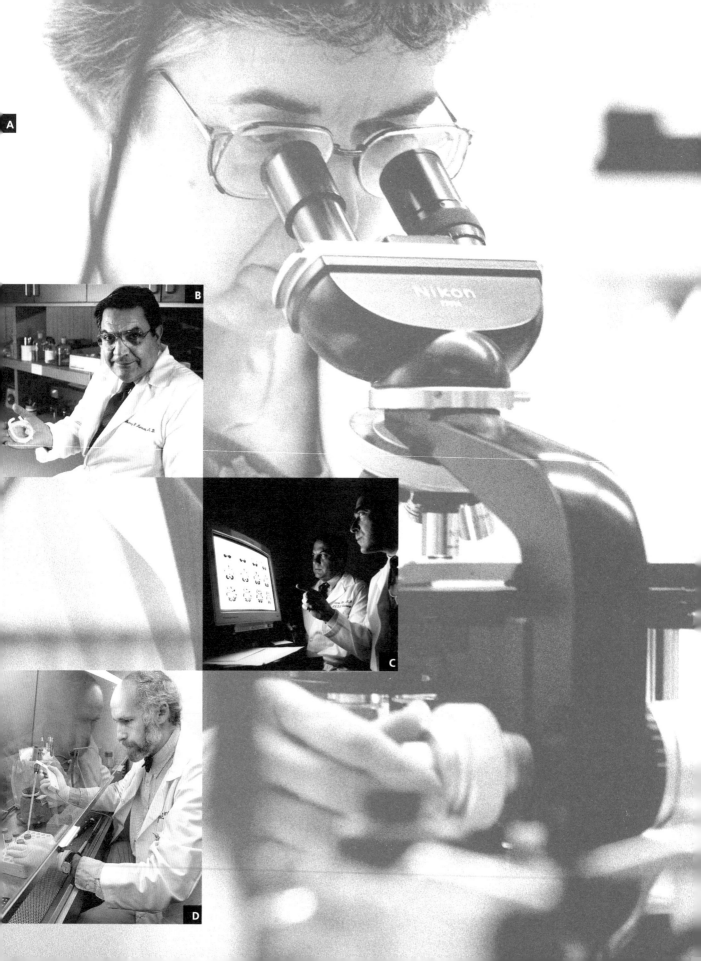

thirteenth largest hospital recipient of federal funding for research, placing it in the top 8 percent of hospitals nationwide.

Nevertheless, federal dollars, while increasing in total, provide only half the funds necessary to support Deaconess research programs, requiring the hospital to pursue alternative funding sources. One means for offsetting the loss in federal funding has been an increase in industry support — an impressive gain given that the corporate dollars available to specific research programs have also diminished, as a result of downsizing, health-care reforms, and an increase in the number of proposals from competing researchers. Private donations have also helped counterbalance the decline in federal funding. Patients and their families have made generous commitments in response to the care received at Deaconess Hospital — care that often evolves directly from laboratory research conducted by Deaconess investigators.

The hospital's current research staff is exploring a myriad of ways to link the research bench to the patient's bedside. In the Department of Medicine, for instance, there are numerous efforts to understand the mechanisms of and therapies for infectious diseases, including AIDS. Jerome Groopman, chief of hematology/oncology and holder of the Recanati Professorship in Immunology at Harvard Medical School, focuses on AIDS/HIV and oversees one of the hospital's busiest laboratories while maintaining a clinical practice of more than 100 patients. Groopman's work in this field dates back to 1980 to his fellowship days at UCLA when he saw his first AIDS patient and subsequently wrote one of the earliest scientific papers describing the disease. Groopman and members of other medical divisions such as infectious disease, pulmonary medicine, dermatology, gastroenterology, and nutrition have made the hospital a leader in AIDS care and research and garnered international recognition for work in this field.

Since 1989 James E. Muller has headed the hospital's cardiology division, succeeding O. Stevens Leland. Muller came to the Deaconess from Brigham and Women's Hospital where he had become widely known for his studies of physiological factors affecting heart disease. Muller launched the hospital's Institute for Prevention of Cardiovascular Disease and recruited other prominent heart researchers to join his team in investigations that explore potential triggers of heart attacks.

DEACONESS HOSPITAL RESEARCH *in the 1990s. The nation's thirteenth largest hospital recipient of federal research funding in 1994, total research awards at the Deaconess currently exceed $11.6 million per annum.*

A SCIENTIST MARY WOOD, *Department of Surgery, conducts research into immunosuppressive therapies that offer transplant patients new prospects for life.*

B DR. ANTHONY P. MONACO, *Department of Surgery, has guided efforts to develop an artificial pancreas that may someday lead to control of diabetes without immunosuppression.*

C DR. THOMAS HILL *(left), Department of Radiological Sciences, and Dr. Russell Vasile, Department of Psychiatry, are collaborating in the use of single photon emission computerized tomography (SPECT) to study the brain and its response to certain treatments for mental health conditions.*

D DR. JEROME E. GROOPMAN, *Department of Medicine, is a pioneer and internationally recognized authority in HIV/AIDS research and care.*

Herbert Benson is well known both within the medical profession and with the general public for his research and writing on the "relaxation response," a term he coined to describe a group of physiologic changes which can be elicited to reduce stress and provide other salutary effects. Benson oversees the hospital's work in behavioral medicine, an interdisciplinary field that bridges medicine, psychology, psychiatry, and nursing. In 1992 Harvard Medical School established the world's first endowed chair in behavioral medicine and named Benson its first occupant. The Mind/Body Medical Institute, headed by Benson, conducts research, teaching, and training in behavioral medicine, not just at the Deaconess but at sites around the country.

The benefits of corporate and private support of research are reflected in the Department of Surgery's Division of Organ Transplantation under the direction of Anthony Monaco. The investigations of research teams led by Monaco and Takashi Maki and by Fritz Bach in the Sandoz Center for Immunobiology concentrate on such problems as ways to circumvent the shortage of human donor organs through artificial organs and xenografts (cross-species transplants) as well as transplantation questions that include the control of organ rejection. Monaco and Maki, for example, are currently developing an artificial pancreas using pig islet cells in the hope of controlling blood sugar in diabetics without immunosuppression.

Under Harvey Goldman, the Department of Pathology has expanded existing research endeavors and made significant clinical contributions to the field of molecular pathology, a new and rapidly expanding subspecialty service which has the capability to advance disease diagnosis and treatment. In addition, the department's residency program, the oldest at the Deaconess, and its nationally recognized Medical Technology School, continue to flourish. The pathology department has expanded its outreach efforts as well. The department currently provides all outpatient lab services for the Boston Visiting Nurses Association and, through its home phlebotomy team, extends care well beyond the hospital's hallways.

Research collaborations among hospital staff are common. In surgical oncology, for example, Glenn Steele has actively pursued studies with Harvey Goldman, among others, in research involving the risk and treatment of gastrointestinal cancers. The pioneering and novel studies in surgery, radiology, and the hospital's cancer biology group have generated new therapies for solid tumors, particularly those of the liver and gastrointestinal tract. Collaborative research efforts between Bruce Bistrian, chief of clinical nutrition, and George Blackburn, chief of surgical nutrition, have led to significant progress in a number of areas including the role of insulin resistance in hypertension, dyslipidemia, Type II diabetes, and gout, and the role of fish oil supplementation in reducing cell proliferation associated with colon cancer.

OVER THE PAST TWO DECADES new technologies in radiological science have been developed while existing ones have been refined to enhance the ability of radiologists to see inside the body. New modalities added to the hospital's radiological armamentarium since 1975 include magnetic resonance imaging (MRI), ultrasound, spiral computer-assisted tomography (CT), single photon emission computer tomography (SPECT), and the new electron beam tomography (EBT) scanner. The advances in imaging hardware enable hospital specialists in radiological science to examine patients, diagnose their disease sooner, and allow for treatment to be implemented at an earlier stage. For patients, the new technology permits conventional imaging to be done faster, more safely, and with better image quality.

Radiology continues to break new ground under its chairman, Melvin E. Clouse, who in 1988 was named a full professor at Harvard Medical School. Clouse has been chairman of the department since 1975 and has successfully turned a fine clinical department into a first-rate academic one as well. Clouse's elevation to a full professorship also recognized his own contributions to interventional and vascular radiology through his work in lymphography, the development of chemoembolization techniques to treat inoperable liver cancer, and studies investigating methods for reducing the cold ischemic effect of preserved livers prior to implantation using magnetic resonance spectroscopy.

Other members of the Department of Radiological Sciences have made important clinical and research contributions. Director of ultrasound Robert Kane and Deaconess urologist Paul Church conducted a nationwide study sponsored by the American Cancer Society on the use of ultrasound in detecting prostate cancer. Kane has also collaborated with Deaconess surgeons in the treatment of liver tumors, changing the way inoperable tumors of the liver are treated using cryoablation (freezing

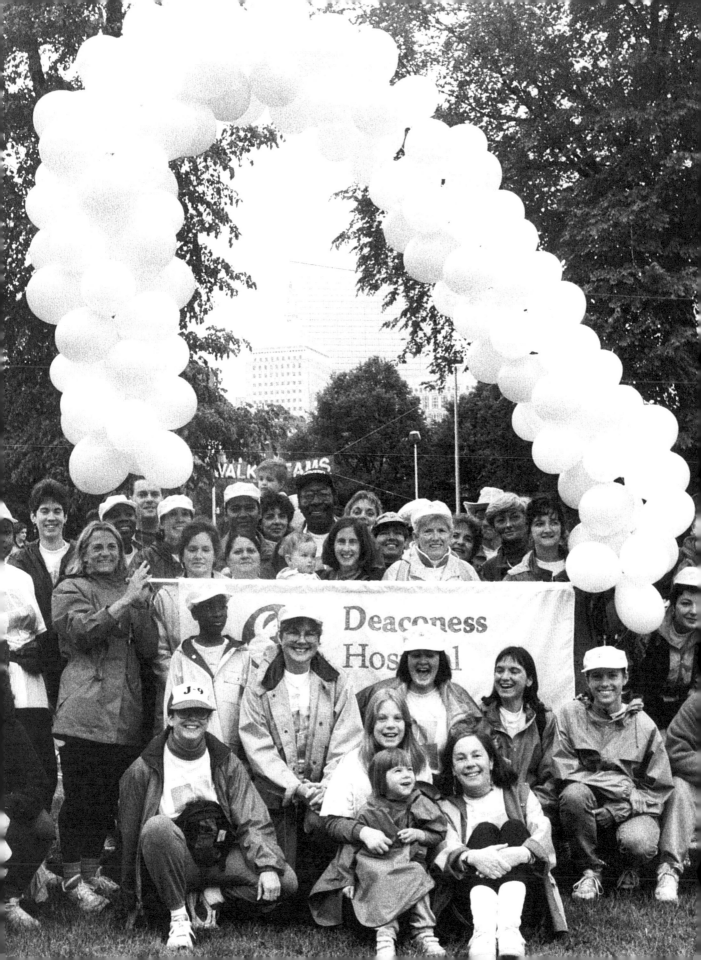

tumors *in situ*). Radiologist Philip Costello has advanced the use of spiral computer-assisted tomography (CT) to determine the patency of coronary artery bypass grafts and to improve imaging of the liver and pancreas. New applications for magnetic resonance imaging angiography as a less invasive technique than standard modalities for imaging coronary artery disease and other applications in cardiology have been pursued by several members of the department, including George Hartnell, who has training and experience in both cardiology and radiology.

Also at the forefront in the use of technology for clinical care has been the Joint Center for Radiation Therapy (JCRT). First under Samuel Hellman's leadership and since 1985 under C. Norman Coleman's, the Joint Center has become one of the leading radiation therapy programs in the country, maintaining a central organization and common treatment philosophy throughout its member institutions, which now include the Deaconess, Beth Israel, Brigham and Women's, and Children's hospitals, and Dana-Farber Cancer Institute. In addition to assuring a consistently high level of clinical care among the institutions, the nature of the Joint Center has permitted collaborative research and training programs that would have been difficult for individual institutions to undertake on their own. An important member of the research and clinical programs of the Joint Center is Paul Busse, the highly regarded clinical chief of radiation oncology at the Deaconess, who has led efforts in the further development of intraoperative radiation treatment.

IN ADDITION TO ITS COMMITMENT to research and clinical excellence, the Deaconess, as a major teaching hospital of Harvard Medical School, is a center for medical training and education. With residency training programs in medicine, pathology, psychiatry, radiation oncology, radiology, and surgery, the hospital attracts a large number of applicants for the available openings. In 1995, for example, more than 650 medical school graduates applied for 30 positions in the hospital's training program in medicine. The Department of Surgery received more than 750 applications for six categorical slots.

The hospital's academic offerings include a new primary-care residency, introduced in 1993 in the Department of Medicine's Division of Internal Medicine, which assures residents extensive patient contact in

Deaconess staff and employees, 1995 AIDS Pledge Walk. From the early deaconesses who provided free care to Boston's indigent to modern affiliations with community-based health facilities such as Roxbury Comprehensive Community Health Center, Inc., the hospital's tradition of community service continues. Through its AIDS Outreach Program, the Deaconess provides educational and training opportunities for a diverse community statewide. One of the hospital's many activities is participation in the annual AIDS Action Committee's Pledge Walk, which Deaconess staff have supported from its inception.

ambulatory care settings. Approximately one quarter of all Harvard Medical School students take their core clerkship in surgery at the Deaconess under the leadership of Frank LoGerfo, George Starkey, and Michael Stone. The highly rated Introduction to Clinical Medicine course, which precedes the core clerkship, is under the guidance of Ronald Silvestri and Lee Simon of the Department of Medicine and Dorothy Freeman and Frank LoGerfo of the Department of Surgery. The hospital's general surgery training program, led by Albert Bothe, is preeminent. A model residency in podiatric surgery and a fellowship in clinical hyperalimentation are nationally recognized. Surgery's continuing education programs have grown in number and popularity. During the 1994-1995 academic year alone, more than 1,000 practicing doctors and others from around the country and the world took courses offered by department members.

FROM THE EARLY DEACONESSES who furnished free care to Boston's poor to present-day outreach activities, compassionate community service has never been confined within the hospital walls. Since its founding, the hospital has endeavored to provide high-quality clinical services to the medically underserved. Under Dick Gaintner's leadership, this commitment has been revitalized to fit the community's changing needs.

Since 1985 one of the hospital's strongest and most dynamic relationships has been with Roxbury Comprehensive Community Health Center, Inc. (RoxComp), which serves the outpatient health-care needs of Roxbury, Mattapan, and Dorchester residents. The relationship began primarily to provide outpatient training for hospital residents, but under the leadership of Gaintner and J. Jacques Carter, the director of the Deaconess/ RoxComp residency program, it has developed into a true sharing of resources and expertise. Hospital residents gain experience in an ambulatory care setting while RoxComp has access to expanded physician services. In 1994 the Deaconess joined RoxComp and New England Baptist and Beth Israel hospitals to establish the Roxbury Heart Center, which provides prevention services and diagnostic testing for populations at risk of developing cardiovascular disease.

As an international leader in the fight against HIV/AIDS, the hospital strives to develop effective treatments, to train clinicians, and to care for people with HIV/AIDS in a compassionate and clinically expert manner.

Through the AIDS Outreach Program, the Deaconess is committed to providing programmatic, educational, and financial support to community-based AIDS-related organizations throughout Massachusetts. The hospital's consultation and service team trains health-care professionals practicing in community settings and provides organizations access to the clinical and research activities of the Deaconess.

In addition, through active participation in such organizations as United Way, the Massachusetts Breast Cancer Coalition, and Project ProTech and the Summer Jobs Program, the Deaconess staff provides educational and training opportunities for the diverse community it serves.

HEALTH CARE FOR THE TWENTY-FIRST CENTURY

To many of those involved in health care, change has never seemed so rapid and relentless as it does in the 1990s. Regionally, as well as nationally, the health-care industry is in a period of substantial restructuring. Changes in the current environment, especially the growth and penetration of managed care and the emergence of new payment mechanisms, have increased competition and created pressure on hospitals to take a broader view of health care and to develop new strategic directions. "This era in health care may prove to be the most dramatic in the history of medicine," observes Dick Gaintner.

The three decades preceding the current health-care revolution were ones of significant growth in the health sector, both in absolute and relative terms. In 1960, 5 percent of the Gross National Product was devoted to health care; by 1993, that figure had risen to 14. Fundamental medical progress and scientific breakthroughs have provided health providers the means to extend lives, but at significant financial cost. Advances in early detection of some diseases such as cancer, the revolution brought about by successful organ transplantation, and the development of vaccines for a variety of diseases from polio to hepatitis have extended both the quality and length of lives. But the financial cost of progress is high and expenditures have escalated. In the 1980s and '90s a fundamental shift from indemnity insurance to health maintenance organizations and managed care was an attempt to control the spiraling costs of health care, one of the legacies of the rapid and widespread accomplishments in

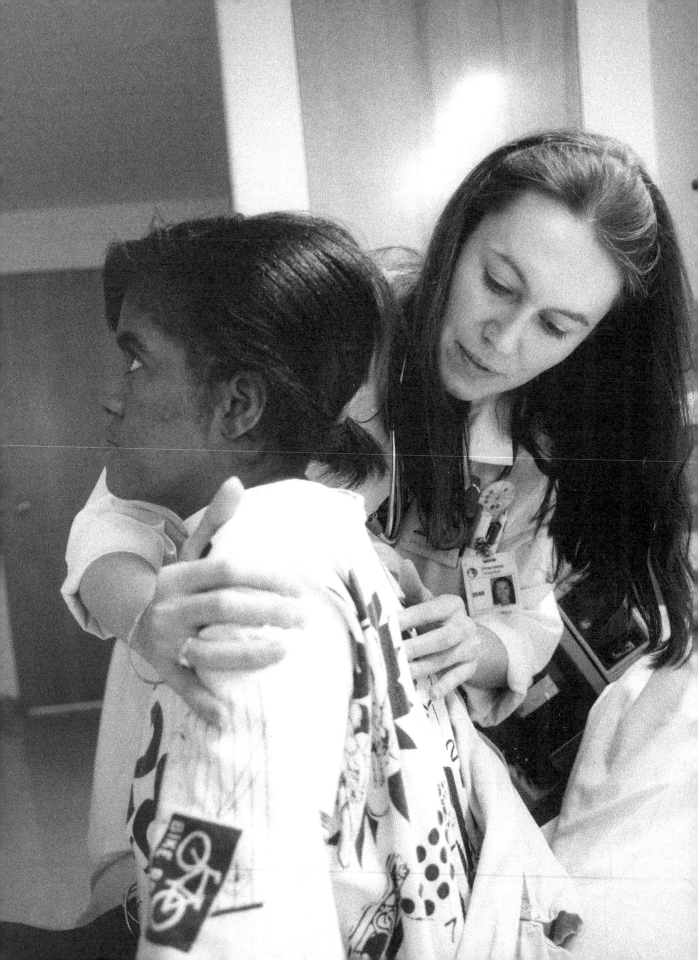

scientific advances. In some respects, tertiary-care facilities such as Deaconess Hospital became the victims of their own success.

ANTICIPATING THE WINDS OF CHANGE, in the late 1980s and early 1990s Deaconess Hospital began developing a strategy to strengthen its position as a specialized tertiary-care facility by establishing ties with community hospitals, physician groups, and health centers that offer complementary services. The goal was to produce the greatest "value" in the health services market by ensuring that patients receive the most appropriate care in the most appropriate setting.

In a sense the seeds for a new Deaconess network were planted in the 1970s, when as a new medical school administrator in Connecticut, Dick Gaintner began working with community hospitals and their staffs to develop regional medical programs. He learned about the needs of community and teaching hospitals and how the two entities are often very different, but also complementary. When Gaintner came to head the Deaconess in 1989, he found a hospital that related very well to community hospitals and community physicians. This approach to delivering care struck a chord with Gaintner, whose experience had fostered enormous respect for health care delivered at the community level. Under Gaintner the informal Deaconess network expanded.

In 1992, Jeffrey R. Kelly, president of The Nashoba Community Hospital, a sixty-three bed hospital in Ayer, Massachusetts, which already had an informal partnership with the Deaconess, approached Gaintner about a more formal arrangement. Gaintner has related that Kelly was concerned about the survival of his hospital, despite its excellence, in the changing health-care environment and wanted to talk of a possible union with the Deaconess. Talk they did and the following year Nashoba Hospital became a subsidiary of the Deaconess's holding corporation and changed its name to Deaconess-Nashoba Hospital.

The success of Deaconess-Nashoba bolstered the strategy Gaintner and the Board of Trustees had already fashioned toward the creation of a formal network of health-care institutions — primary, secondary, and tertiary — each of which would provide high-quality care appropriate to its own setting. What eventually emerged was Pathway Health Network. The network philosophy offers patients access to

DEACONESS THIRD-YEAR MEDICAL RESIDENT DR. JOANNA PREIBISZ AND HER PATIENT PHYLLIS MONTEIRO, 1992. As a major teaching hospital of Harvard Medical School, the Deaconess is dedicated to cultivating the talent of young physicians. With training programs in medicine, pathology, psychiatry, radiation oncology, radiology, and surgery, the hospital provides an important foundation in both the art and the science of medicine.

physicians and community hospitals as well as to highly trained specialists at academic medical centers while preserving the character and internal efficiency of the individual institutions. The goal of Pathway Health, according to its leadership, is "to provide optimum, cost-effective care for patients while positioning network members to take advantage of the emerging managed-care market."

Instrumental in the creation of Pathway Health Network was the affiliation of New England Baptist Hospital. In the late 1980s New England Baptist Hospital had developed a strategic plan to emphasize several specialties while articulating a desire to form an alliance with one of Boston's teaching hospitals to complement the services it offered. Founded in 1893, the Baptist had a parallel history to the slightly younger Deaconess, with an excellent diploma nursing school, a strong tradition of patient care, and a past close relationship with the Lahey Clinic. The Baptist had considered joining with the Deaconess before. Indeed, the Deaconess pathology department had long provided services to the Baptist, while many members of the two hospitals' medical staffs, particularly in cardiology, held joint appointments. The Baptist was a specialty-referral institution with highly regarded programs in the treatment of musculoskeletal disorders and orthopedics. According to Baptist President and Chief Executive Officer Raymond McAfoose, the Deaconess affiliation was chosen because it enabled the Baptist to retain its own identity, license, medical staff, board of trustees, and endowment while becoming "part of a system that would allow us to collaborate, rationalize services, save money through various joint ventures, and just become stronger." On July 1, 1994, New England Baptist formally joined Pathway Health Network.

One of the first examples of the synergies that can be created through network collaboration was the establishment of New England Bone & Joint Institute at the Baptist, a union of the Deaconess's clinical and research programs in rheumatology under the leadership of Steven Goldring, and the Baptist's expertise in diagnosis and treatment of orthopedic conditions. A center of excellence program for Pathway Health Network, the Institute offers a continuum of care for persons with, or at risk for, limitation in mobility and/or bone, muscle, or joint pain.

With the network in place, other area institutions began to look for a solution to the "survival-of-the-fittest" race without a loss of autonomy and character. In 1993 the Town of Needham (Massachusetts) wanted to get out of the hospital business and was looking for a buyer for the municipal Glover Memorial Hospital. The Deaconess won a competitive bidding process because, as Glover President and Chief Executive Officer John Dalton recalls, "this was the only opportunity for Glover that could preserve both the community medical staff and a community institution." On July 1, 1994, Deaconess-Glover Hospital became official. By 1995 WalthamWeston Hospital and Medical Center was also a Pathway Health affiliate with a new name — Deaconess-Waltham Hospital.

In addition, the network maintains programmatic, clinical, and academic relationships with other hospitals, health centers, and physician groups. And Pathway Health continues to uphold a commitment to academic and clinical excellence personified by Deaconess Hospital itself as well as New England Bone & Joint Institute at New England Baptist.

The creation of Pathway Health brought about changes in the administration of both Deaconess Hospital and the growing network. Al Washko moved up to become president and chief executive officer of the Deaconess as Dick Gaintner assumed a full-time role as president and chief executive officer of Pathway Health Network. Similarly, Gregg Stone succeeded John Hamill as chairman of the hospital board of directors as Hamill moved over to chair the network board.

BUILDING FOR THE FUTURE

With its staff and programs flourishing and with its financial balance sheet restored to health, in 1989 the Deaconess was able to revive plans for physical rejuvenation. Although Payette Associates had served as architects on the preliminary proposal in the mid-1980s, Gaintner decided to open up the design selection process. In April of 1990, Shepley Bulfinch Richardson and Abbott, the renowned Boston firm which had designed several of the Deaconess's buildings in the past, was selected as architects of the hospital's new Clinical Center, which at 330,000 square feet is the largest building project in the hospital's history.

These new facilities and improvements were expensive — the Clinical Center alone cost $135 million. In 1992, the Board of Trustees launched a $35 million capital campaign, with $10 million earmarked for the Clinical Center and $25 million for research consolidation. Among

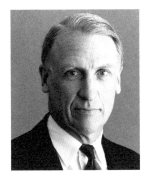

JOHN P. HAMILL, 1993.
A member of the hospital's Board of Trustees since 1985, Hamill served as chairman from 1991 until 1995, when he assumed the chairmanship of Pathway Health Network.

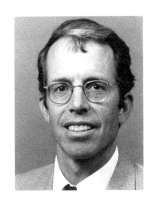

R. GREGG STONE, 1995.
A Deaconess corporator and trustee for over a decade, Stone became chairman of the hospital board in 1995.

the individuals and groups providing substantial support for the fund-raising effort were members of the hospital's senior management team, physician practice plans, employees, and nursing alumni. The Friends of the Deaconess, which had raised $201 in its first year during the Depression, committed its membership to raising a total of $500,000.

The Deaconess's finances for such an endeavor had been strengthened by the sale of two assets. In anticipation of its new research facility, in 1992 the Deaconess sold the Shields Warren Laboratory building to Dana-Farber Cancer Institute. This transaction generated about $4 million in cash and allowed the hospital use of the space through a lease extending for seven years.

But it was the sale of Deaconess Home Health Care Corporation (DHHCC) that brought a much larger yield. Founded in 1984 during MacLure's presidency, with strong backing from Dick Lee, DHHCC provided high-quality, cost-effective care and supplies to patients in their homes. The corporation emphasized intravenous and infusion therapy and respiratory care and served patients throughout New England. Under its president, Richard Baptista, and with significant contributions from George Blackburn and his team in surgical nutrition, DHHCC had experienced enormous growth; revenues grew by 350 percent in the four years ending in 1990. Gregg Stone and James Morgan, astute venture capitalists on the Deaconess board, argued that the time was right to get out of this business. Reimbursement practices were changing and the hospital's board and management were focusing on building a health-care network and could not devote appropriate attention to this as well. In 1992 certain assets of DHHCC were sold to a private company, with a net gain to the parent corporation of about $25 million, a remarkable achievement considering how recently the enterprise had been created.

WITH FUND-RAISING EFFORTS WELL UNDER WAY, attention was turned to planning the hospital's new facilities. The design requirements for the new Clinical Center were prodigious. Trustee Vincent Vappi, a leading builder himself and a strong proponent of plant revitalization, expertly chaired the board's building committee. In the spring of 1992, the venerable Harris Hall was torn down and the foundation laid for the new structure. Progress was rapid; the Clinical Center opened in early 1995, well ahead of schedule.

The seven-story structure, with its granite, brick, and glass facade, gives the Deaconess a new presence on Brookline Avenue. The Clinical Center contains seventeen state-of-the-art operating rooms, sophisticated intensive care units, efficiently located imaging suites, conference rooms and classrooms with video conferencing and telemedicine capabilities, computerized workstations and fiber-optic communication lines, and an expanded emergency room.

The Clinical Center marks the first stage of the hospital's current building program, which also includes consolidated research space. The proximity of research to clinical services is essential for the Deaconess. Consolidated space will enable hospital staff to take full advantage of interdisciplinary collaboration. It will also reduce redundancies in equipment, purchasing, material, and human resources. In addition, the Deaconess has proceeded with the renovation of some of its existing facilities, including patient rooms, a new secure unit in psychiatry, elevator modernization, and updating of physician practice areas.

WITH THE COMPLETION OF THE CLINICAL CENTER, the nearly century-old Deaconess Hospital begins a new chapter in its history. Just as the original fourteen-bed infirmary was founded to unite science and kindliness in the war against disease, so, too, the Deaconess Hospital of today has committed its resources to care for the sickest of patients with both competence and compassion.

*Dr. Shields Warren,
1977. For five decades,
Warren personified
Deaconess medicine.
Uniting a natural
curiosity and scientific
expertise with a genuine
concern for patients,
Warren practiced and
inspired in others the skill
and compassion that
have come to represent the
essence of Deaconess
Hospital.*

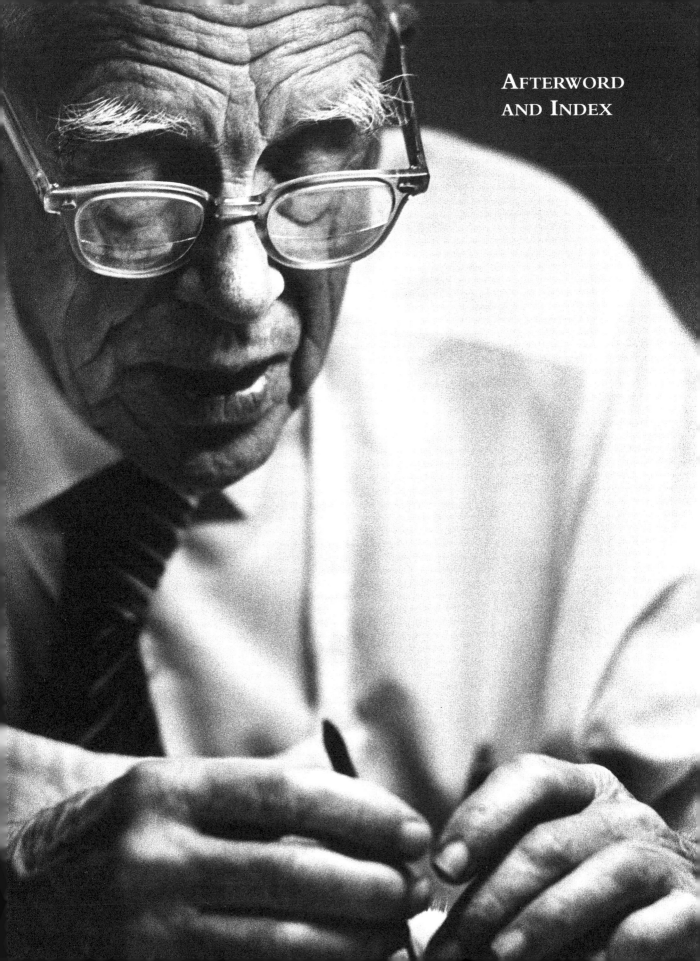

Afterword

Historians have no particular ability or skill at predicting the future. It has sometimes been said, they have challenge enough in predicting the past. Students of history, however, can sometimes derive lessons, both cautionary and inspirational, from what has gone before. Readers are encouraged to draw their own lessons from this account, but a few observations are now offered for general consideration.

One is that the Deaconess has always been a dynamic institution. Although there is a natural tendency to see the hospital's past as static and to see its current situation as fraught with uncertainty and change, the Deaconess has, in fact, changed constantly over time. The Deaconess of 1930 was as different from the Deaconess of 1910 as the Deaconess of 1990 was from the hospital of 1970.

The path has not always been easy. There have been moments of great uncertainty along the way: Would there ever be enough money to complete the early Deaconess Building? Would the hospital survive the Depression? How would it cope with the staff shortages of World War II? How would it manage after the Lahey Clinic left? Could it evolve as a successful teaching hospital?

Alongside this change and uncertainty, there have always been certain continuities in what might be called the Deaconess institutional culture. Thanks primarily to its founding by deaconesses and to the strong nursing tradition that took root under them, especially through its excellent hospital nursing school, the Deaconess has always highly valued patient care. After all, it was the quality and dedication of the nursing staff that first attracted outstanding doctors and kept them at the Deaconess over many years. That long-standing tradition of patient care remains alive today.

Science constitutes another continuity. Although the Deaconess was not until quite recently a major teaching hospital, there has been a long tradition of clinical scientific investigation and excellence dating back to Elliott Joslin, Frank Lahey, and Shields Warren. Specialty training and fellowship programs were introduced at the Deaconess more than sixty years ago. Thus, while science and teaching have expanded

216

exponentially in the last fifteen years, they were threads in the hospital's fabric long before that.

A third continuity can be found in the high quality of the Deaconess's management and board. The hospital has been fortunate to have been well and capably administered, managed, and led over the years — by, among others, Mary Lunn, Adeliza Betts, Warren Cook, Don Lowry, Laurie MacLure, and Dick Gaintner. Just four individuals, Cook, Lowry, MacLure, and Gaintner, served as the Deaconess's chief administrative officer over a sixty-nine-year period, a remarkable record of leadership stability. The Deaconess has also had many community members who have given freely of their time, energy, and wisdom as volunteers on the hospital board, with many of them serving long tenures.

Whatever challenges and difficulties await, the Deaconess should derive strength and confidence from its rich, dynamic, and not always easy past. The hospital's institutional culture and its long-standing dedication to providing excellent patient care together with the finest contemporary medical science should stand the Deaconess in good stead for a second century of distinguished service.

INDEX

Italicized page numbers denote photographs

About the Author

Historian Carl M. Brauer has written books, articles, essays, and reviews on a wide range of subjects in twentieth-century America. He has also edited documentary collections and memoirs. After earning his Ph.D. in American history from Harvard University in 1973, Brauer spent the next fifteen years in academic life. Since 1989 he has been an independent historian. His other books include *John F. Kennedy and the Second Reconstruction* (1977), *Presidential Transitions: Eisenhower Through Reagan* (1986), *Ropes & Gray, 1865–1990* (1991), and *The Man Who Built Washington: A Life of John McShain* (in press). Brauer lives in Belmont, Massachusetts, where he also maintains a professional office.